28-DAY TRANSFORMATIVE ENDOMORPH DIET AND EXERCISE PLAN

A Science-Backed Guide with Personalized Meal Plans, Delicious Recipes, and Tailored Exercise Plan to Boost Metabolism, Burn Fat and Lose Weight.

TIMOTHY A. GWIN

Copyright Page

TABLE OF CONTENTS

Introduction

- Understanding your Body Type — 6
- Importance of a Customized Plan — 7
- Effective Exercise Regimen — 7

Endomorph

- What is an Endomorph? — 10
- Genetic Factors — 10
- Common Misconceptions — 11

Metabolism and Endomorph

- Characteristics and Metabolic Traits — 14
- How Metabolism Affects Weight — 15

Nutrition For Endomorphs

- Macronutrients — 16
- Micronutrients — 17
- Importance and Benefits of Hydration — 18

- **Food to Include & Avoid For Endomorphs** — 20

Designing Your Meal Plan

- Daily Calorie Needs — 26
- Meal Timing and Frequency — 27
- **28-Day Meal Plan** — 30

- Vegetable Omelette 34
- Greek Yogurt Parfait 35
- Avocado & Egg Breakfast Bowl 36
- Protein Smoothie Recipe 37
- Chia Seed Pudding 38
- Keto Breakfast Burrito 39
- Stuffed Bell Peppers 40
- Healthy Cauliflower Hash Browns 41

- Homemade Mushroom & Barley Soup 42
- Tuna Salad in Lettuce Wraps 43
- Beef & Broccoli Stir-Fry 44
- Grilled Chicken Salad 45
- Eggplant Parmesan 46
- Chickpea & Veggie Salad 47
- Grilled Shrimp Tacos 48
- Spaghetti Squash with Turkey Bolognese 50
- Grilled Portobello Mushrooms 52
- Herbed pork Tenderloin 53
- Chicken Fajita Bowl 54
- Almond-Crusted Tilapia 55
- Meaty Muffins 56
- Endo Guacamole 57
- Endo Parmesan Asparagus 58

- Turnip Chips   59
- Pear Slices with Ricotta   60
- Cucumber Slice with Tzatziki   61
- Hard Boiled Eggs   62
- Air Popped Popcorn   63

- **Exercise For Endomorphs**   64
- **Importance of Consistency**   65
- **Balancing Cardio & Strength Training**   66
- **Rest and Recovery**   67
- **List of Exercises**   68
- **Tips for success**   70
- **28-Day Exercise Plan**   72

WELCOME TO YOUR ENDOMORPH JOURNEY

Embarking on a journey to better health and fitness is an exciting and transformative experience. If you've identified yourself as an endomorph, you're in the right place. Understanding your body type is crucial for developing an effective and personalized approach to fitness and nutrition. This guide will provide you with comprehensive insights into your unique body type, the importance of a customized plan, and an overview of how this book will support you every step of the way.

UNDERSTANDING YOUR BODY TYPE

Endomorphs are characterized by a tendency to store fat more easily than other body types. This means that you might find it challenging to lose weight and maintain a lean physique. However, this body type also has its advantages, such as the potential for significant muscle mass and strength. Here are some key traits of endomorphs:

- **Body Shape:** Endomorphs often have a rounder, softer body shape with wider hips and a higher percentage of body fat.
- **Metabolism:** Generally, endomorphs have a slower metabolism, which can contribute to easier weight gain and more difficulty with weight loss.
- **Muscle Mass:** Despite the higher fat storage, endomorphs can build muscle relatively easily, which can be advantageous for strength training.
- **Fat Distribution:** Fat tends to be distributed around the abdomen, hips, and thighs.

IMPORTANCE OF A CUSTOMIZED PLAN

A one-size-fits-all approach to fitness and nutrition often leads to frustration and suboptimal results, especially for endomorphs. Here's why a customized plan is essential:

Tailored Nutrition

Endomorphs benefit significantly from a nutrition plan that supports their slower metabolism and tendency to store fat. Key elements include:

- **Macronutrient Balance:** Emphasizing higher protein intake to support muscle maintenance and lower carbohydrate intake to manage insulin levels and reduce fat storage.
- **Meal Timing:** Strategically timing meals to regulate blood sugar levels and metabolism. For instance, consuming smaller, more frequent meals can prevent overeating and spikes in blood sugar.
- **Healthy Fats:** Including sources of healthy fats can help control cravings and provide sustained energy.

Effective Exercise Regimen

Exercise plays a critical role in managing weight and building muscle for endomorphs. A well-rounded plan should incorporate:

- **Strength Training:** Focus on compound movements that target multiple muscle groups, enhancing muscle growth and boosting metabolism.
- **Cardiovascular Exercise:** Incorporating high-intensity interval training (HIIT) can be particularly effective for fat loss while preserving muscle mass.
- **Flexibility and Recovery:** Stretching and proper recovery techniques to prevent injury and maintain muscle health.

Lifestyle Adjustments

In addition to diet and exercise, lifestyle factors such as sleep, stress management, and hydration are crucial. Endomorphs should prioritize:

- **Quality Sleep:** Adequate sleep is essential for metabolic health and recovery.
- **Stress Management**: Chronic stress can lead to hormonal imbalances that promote fat storage, so practices like mindfulness and relaxation techniques are beneficial.
- **Hydration:** Proper hydration supports metabolism and overall health.

WHAT IS AN ENDOMORPH?

An endomorph is one of the three somatotypes, a classification system developed by American psychologist William Sheldon in the 1940s. Somatotypes categorize human bodies into three broad types based on their build and composition: ectomorph, mesomorph, and endomorph. Endomorphs are characterized by a higher percentage of body fat, wider waists, and larger bone structures. They tend to gain weight easily and may find it challenging to lose fat. Their metabolism is often slower compared to other body types, making it more difficult for them to burn calories efficiently.

Key characteristics of endomorphs include:

- A soft, round body with a higher fat percentage.
- A tendency to store fat, particularly in the abdominal area.
- A broader waist and hips.
- Shorter limbs relative to their torso.
- A less defined muscle structure.
- A naturally slower metabolic rate.

GENETIC FACTORS

Genetics play a crucial role in determining an individual's somatotype. Endomorphs typically inherit their body composition from their parents. Several genetic factors contribute to the traits associated with endomorph:

- **Metabolism:** Endomorphs generally have a slower basal metabolic rate (BMR), which is the rate at which the body uses energy while at rest. This lower BMR can be attributed to genetic variations that influence how efficiently the body converts food into energy.

- **Fat Storage and Distribution**: Genetic predisposition affects how and where the body stores fat. Endomorphs are more likely to have genes that promote fat storage, especially in the abdominal region. This is partly due to the way their bodies process and store energy.

- **Muscle and Bone Structure**: The wider bone structure and larger frame typical of endomorphs are also influenced by genetics. These physical characteristics can affect the body's overall shape and propensity to gain or lose weight.

- **Hormonal Influence**: Hormones play a significant role in determining body composition. Endomorphs may have hormonal profiles that favor fat storage. For instance, they might have higher levels of insulin, which promotes fat storage, or lower levels of thyroid hormones, which can slow down metabolism.

COMMON MISCONCEPTIONS

Several misconceptions surround the concept of endomorphs, often leading to misunderstandings about weight management and fitness for individuals with this body type.

- **Endomorphs Can't Lose Weight:** One of the most common misconceptions is that endomorphs are unable to lose weight effectively. While it may be more challenging for endomorphs to shed pounds due to their slower metabolism, it is not impossible. With a well-structured diet and exercise regimen tailored to their specific needs, endomorphs can achieve significant weight loss and improve their body composition.

- **Endomorphs Are Lazy:** Another myth is that endomorphs are inherently lazy or unmotivated. This stereotype overlooks the genetic and physiological factors that contribute to their body type. Many endomorphs are active and committed to their fitness goals, but they may need to work harder and longer to see results compared to their ectomorphic or mesomorphic counterparts.

- **All Endomorphs Are Unhealthy:** Being an endomorph does not automatically equate to being unhealthy. While endomorphs may have a higher body fat percentage, health is determined by various factors, including diet, exercise, and overall lifestyle. Many endomorphs maintain excellent health through balanced nutrition and regular physical activity.

- **Endomorphs is Fixed and Unchangeable:** Some people believe that being an endomorph is a permanent state that cannot be altered. While genetic predisposition plays a significant role, individuals can influence their body composition through lifestyle changes. Diet, exercise, and other factors can significantly impact an endomorph's ability to manage weight and improve fitness levels.

- **Endomorphs Can't Build Muscle:** While endomorphs may have a harder time losing fat, they often have an advantage when it comes to building muscle. Their larger frame and bone structure can support more muscle mass. With proper strength training and nutrition, endomorphs can develop a muscular and toned physique.

METABOLISM AND ENDOMORPHS

Metabolism refers to the sum of all chemical processes that occur within a living organism in order to maintain life. These processes include catabolism (the breakdown of molecules to obtain energy) and anabolism (the synthesis of all compounds needed by the cells). The rate at which these processes occur is known as the **metabolic rate**.

- **Basal Metabolic Rate (BMR):** This is the amount of energy expended while at rest in a neutrally temperate environment, in the post-absorptive state (i.e., the digestive system is inactive). It accounts for about 60-75% of the total daily energy expenditure in most people.

- **Total Daily Energy Expenditure (TDEE):** This is the total amount of calories burned in a day, including BMR, physical activity, and the thermic effect of food (the energy required for digestion, absorption, and disposal of ingested nutrients).

ENDOMORPHS: CHARACTERISTICS AND METABOLIC TRAITS

Endomorphs are one of the three primary body types (somatotypes). The other two types are ectomorphs and mesomorphs. Endomorphs typically have the following characteristics:

- **Body Shape:** They tend to have a rounder and softer physique with a higher percentage of body fat.
- **Bone Structure:** Endomorphs usually have a larger bone structure, broader hips, and a wider waist.
- **Fat Distribution:** They store fat easily, often in the abdominal area, but can also accumulate it around the hips and thighs.
- **Muscle Mass:** While they can build muscle relatively easily, their higher body fat percentage often masks muscle definition.

HOW METABOLISM AFFECTS WEIGHT

Metabolism plays a critical role in determining body weight. The balance between calorie intake and energy expenditure dictates whether an individual gains, loses, or maintains weight. Here's how metabolism impacts weight:

- **Caloric Balance:** Weight gain occurs when calorie intake exceeds calorie expenditure. Conversely, weight loss happens when calorie expenditure surpasses calorie intake.

- **Metabolic Rate:** Individuals with a higher metabolic rate burn more calories at rest and during activity, making it easier to maintain or lose weight. Those with a lower metabolic rate, typical in endomorphs, burn fewer calories and may struggle more with weight management.

- **Hormonal Influence:** Hormones such as thyroid hormones, insulin, and cortisol significantly influence metabolism. Thyroid hormones regulate the metabolic rate, insulin controls blood glucose levels and fat storage, and cortisol, the stress hormone, can lead to increased fat accumulation, especially in the abdominal area.

NUTRITION FOR ENDOMORPHS

Endomorphs are individuals with a body type characterized by a higher percentage of body fat, broader waistlines, and a tendency to gain weight easily. Proper nutrition is essential for managing weight and optimizing health for endomorphs. This includes a balanced intake of macronutrients, micronutrients, and adequate hydration.

MACRONUTRIENTS: PROTEIN, CARBS, AND FATS

PROTEIN

- **Importance:** Protein is crucial for muscle repair, growth, and maintenance. For endomorphs, higher protein intake can aid in maintaining muscle mass while promoting fat loss. It also helps in increasing satiety, reducing overall caloric intake.
- **Sources:** Lean meats (chicken, turkey), fish, eggs, dairy products (Greek yogurt, cottage cheese), legumes (beans, lentils), and plant-based proteins (tofu, tempeh, quinoa).
- **Recommendations:** Endomorphs should aim for about 0.8 to 1 gram of protein per pound of body weight. For someone weighing 150 pounds, this translates to 120 to 150 grams of protein per day.

CARBOHYDRATES

- **Importance:** Carbohydrates are the primary energy source for the body. However, for endomorphs, who are prone to insulin sensitivity and fat storage, the type and timing of carbohydrate intake are crucial.
- **Sources:** Focus on complex carbohydrates like whole grains (brown rice, quinoa, oats), vegetables, and legumes. These provide sustained energy and are less likely to spike blood sugar levels compared to simple carbs.

- **Recommendations:** Carbohydrate intake should be moderate, constituting about 30-40% of daily calories. Prioritizing complex carbs and limiting simple sugars can help manage weight and improve insulin sensitivity.

FATS

- **Importance:** Fats are essential for hormone production, cell membrane integrity, and the absorption of fat-soluble vitamins (A, D, E, K). Healthy fats can also aid in satiety and prevent overeating.
- **Sources:** Healthy fats include avocados, nuts, seeds, olive oil, and fatty fish (salmon, mackerel).
- **Recommendations:** Fat intake should be around 25-35% of daily calories. Emphasize unsaturated fats while limiting saturated and trans fats.

MICRONUTRIENTS: VITAMINS AND MINERALS

VITAMINS

- **Importance:** Vitamins are essential for numerous biochemical processes, including energy production, immune function, and cellular repair.

- **Vitamin D:** Important for bone health and immune function. Endomorphs may need supplementation, especially if they have limited sun exposure.
- **B Vitamins:** Crucial for energy metabolism. Include a variety of sources like whole grains, meats, and leafy greens.
- **Vitamin C:** Supports the immune system and acts as an antioxidant. Found in citrus fruits, strawberries, and bell peppers.

MINERALS

- **Importance:** Minerals play critical roles in bone health, fluid balance, and muscle function.
- **Calcium:** Necessary for bone health. Sources include dairy products, leafy greens, and fortified plant milks.
- **Magnesium:** Involved in over 300 biochemical reactions, including muscle and nerve function. Found in nuts, seeds, and whole grains.
- **Iron:** Essential for oxygen transport in the blood. Sources include red meat, beans, and spinach.

IMPORTANCE OF HYDRATION

Hydration is vital for all body types, including endomorphs. Proper hydration supports digestion, nutrient absorption, and overall metabolic function.

BENEFITS

- **Metabolic Efficiency:** Water is crucial for metabolic processes. Dehydration can slow down metabolism, making it harder to lose weight.
- **Appetite Control:** Often, thirst is mistaken for hunger. Drinking enough water can help control appetite and prevent overeating.
- **Exercise Performance:** Hydration is essential for maintaining energy levels and performance during workouts. Endomorphs, who may need to engage in regular physical activity to manage weight, should pay special attention to their water intake.

RECOMMENDATIONS:

- Aim for at least 8-10 glasses (64-80 ounces) of water per day. Individual needs may vary based on activity level, climate, and overall health.

- Increase water intake during and after exercise to compensate for fluid lost through sweat.
- Incorporate hydrating foods like fruits (watermelon, oranges) and vegetables (cucumbers, celery) into the diet.

For endomorphs, a well-balanced diet focusing on appropriate macronutrient ratios, sufficient micronutrient intake, and proper hydration is essential. Prioritizing protein, moderating carbohydrate intake, and incorporating healthy fats can help manage weight and improve overall health. Ensuring adequate vitamins and minerals supports metabolic functions and general well-being, while proper hydration enhances metabolic efficiency, appetite control, and physical performance.

FOODS TO INCLUDE AND AVOID FOR ENDOMORPHS

Endomorphs are characterized by a higher propensity to store fat, a rounder body shape, and a slower metabolism. People with this body type often find it challenging to lose weight and may gain weight easily if their diet is not well- managed.

BEST FOODS FOR ENDOMORPHS

To manage their weight and optimize their health, endomorphs should focus on a diet that is balanced but slightly skewed towards certain macronutrients.

Proteins:

- **Lean Meats:** Chicken breast, turkey, and lean cuts of beef or pork provide high-quality protein without excessive fat.
- **Fish:** Particularly fatty fish like salmon, mackerel, and sardines, which are rich in omega-3 fatty acids that can help reduce inflammation and improve metabolism.
- **Eggs:** A great source of protein and essential nutrients, eggs can be included in various meals.
- **Legumes:** Beans, lentils, and chickpeas offer both protein and fiber, helping with satiety and digestive health.

Vegetables:

- **Leafy Greens:** Spinach, kale, and Swiss chard are low in calories and high in essential vitamins and minerals.
- **Cruciferous Vegetables:** Broccoli, cauliflower, and Brussels sprouts are nutrient-dense and support detoxification processes.
- **Colorful Veggies:** Peppers, carrots, and tomatoes provide a variety of vitamins and antioxidants.

Fruits:

- **Berries:** Blueberries, strawberries, and raspberries are low in sugar and high in fiber and antioxidants.
- **Citrus Fruits:** Oranges, lemons, and grapefruits are good sources of vitamin C and fiber.
- **Apples and Pears:** High in fiber, these fruits can help with fullness and provide steady energy.

Whole Grains:

- **Quinoa:** A high-protein grain that is also gluten-free and packed with nutrients.
- **Brown Rice:** Provides sustained energy and fiber, supporting digestive health.
- **Oats:** Great for breakfast, oats are high in soluble fiber, which helps control blood sugar levels.

Healthy Fats:

- **Avocados:** Rich in monounsaturated fats and fiber, avocados support heart health and satiety.
- **Nuts and Seeds:** Almonds, chia seeds, and flaxseeds provide healthy fats, fiber, and protein.
- **Olive Oil:** A staple of the Mediterranean diet, olive oil is rich in heart-healthy monounsaturated fats.

Dairy:

- **Low-Fat Yogurt:** Offers protein and probiotics, beneficial for gut health.
- **Cottage Cheese:** High in protein and low in fat, it's a versatile dairy option.
- **Milk:** Preferably low-fat or skim, milk provides essential nutrients like calcium and vitamin D.

FOODS TO MINIMIZE OR AVOID

Endomorphs should minimize or avoid foods that can contribute to fat storage and metabolic slowdowns.

Refined Carbohydrates:
- **White Bread and Pastries:** These offer little nutritional value and can spike blood sugar levels.
- **Sugary Cereals:** Often high in added sugars and low in fiber, they can lead to energy crashes.
- **White Pasta and Rice:** Opt for whole grain versions to get more fiber and nutrients.

Sugary Foods and Drinks:
- **Soda and Sweetened Beverages:** High in empty calories and sugars, they can lead to weight gain and metabolic issues.
- **Candy and Sweets:** These provide excessive sugar without any nutritional benefits.
- **Desserts:** Cakes, cookies, and ice cream should be occasional treats due to their high sugar and fat content.

Processed Foods:
- **Processed Meats:** Sausages, hot dogs, and deli meats often contain high levels of unhealthy fats and sodium.
- **Ready-to-Eat Meals:** These can be high in unhealthy fats, sugars, and sodium.
- **Snack Foods:** Chips, crackers, and similar snacks usually contain refined carbs and unhealthy fats.

High-Fat Foods:

- **Fried Foods:** French fries, fried chicken, and other deep-fried items can add excessive calories and unhealthy fats.
- **High-Fat Dairy:** Full-fat cheese, cream, and butter should be limited due to their high saturated fat content.
- **Certain Oils:** Avoid trans fats and limit saturated fats, opting for healthier oils like olive or avocado oil instead.

UNDERSTANDING FOOD LABELS

Reading and understanding food labels can help endomorphs make healthier choices and avoid foods that may hinder their weight management goals.

Serving Size:

- Always check the serving size first. Many packaged foods contain multiple servings, and consuming more than the serving size listed will increase the intake of all listed nutrients, including calories, fats, and sugars.

Calories:

- Pay attention to the number of calories per serving and how they fit into your daily caloric needs.

Macronutrients:

- Total Fat: Look for the types of fat included. Aim for foods low in saturated and trans fats.
- Carbohydrates: Focus on the amount of dietary fiber and sugars. Higher fiber is better, and lower added sugars are preferable.
- Protein: A higher protein content can help with satiety and muscle maintenance.

Micronutrients:

- Check for essential vitamins and minerals like vitamin D, calcium, iron, and potassium. These are often under-consumed nutrients.

Ingredient List:

- Ingredients are listed in descending order by weight. Aim for foods with whole, recognizable ingredients. Avoid products where sugar or unhealthy fats appear high on the list.

Daily Value Percentages:

- These percentages help you understand how a serving of the food contributes to your daily nutrient needs based on a 2,000-calorie diet. Aim for lower percentages of saturated fats, added sugars, and sodium, and higher percentages of fiber, vitamins, and minerals.

For endomorphs, managing diet is crucial to balance metabolism, control weight, and maintain overall health. Focusing on nutrient-dense foods like lean proteins, vegetables, fruits, whole grains, and healthy fats, while minimizing refined carbs, sugary foods, processed items, and unhealthy fats, can make a significant difference. Additionally, understanding and using food labels can guide better food choices, supporting a healthier lifestyle tailored to the endomorph body type.

DESIGNING YOUR MEAL PLAN

DAILY CALORIC NEEDS

Understanding Caloric Needs for Endomorphs

Endomorphs typically have a slower metabolism, which means they need to be more vigilant about their caloric intake to avoid weight gain. The basal metabolic rate (BMR) for endomorphs is generally lower than that of ectomorphs and mesomorphs, necessitating careful caloric management.

Calculating Daily Caloric Needs

- **Basal Metabolic Rate (BMR):** The BMR can be calculated using the Mifflin-St Jeor Equation:
  - **For men:**
  - BMR=10 × weight in kg + 6.25 × height in cm−5 × age in years + 5BMR= 10 × weight in kg + 6.25 × height in cm−5 × age in years + 5
  - **For women:**
  - BMR= 10 × weight in kg + 6.25 × height in cm−5 × age in years−161BMR= 10 × weight in kg + 6.25×height in cm−5 × age in years−161
- **Total Daily Energy Expenditure (TDEE):** The TDEE takes into account the BMR and the level of physical activity:
  - **Sedentary (little or no exercise):** TDEE = BMR × 1.2
  - **Lightly active (light exercise/sports 1-3 days/week):** TDEE = BMR × 1.375
  - **Moderately active (moderate exercise/sports 3-5 days/week):** TDEE = BMR × 1.55
  - **Very active (hard exercise/sports 6-7 days a week):** TDEE = BMR × 1.725
  - **Super active (very hard exercise, physical job, or training twice a day):** TDEE = BMR × 1.9

Adjusting Caloric Intake for Weight Goals

- **Weight Loss:** Create a caloric deficit by reducing daily intake by 500-1000 calories from the TDEE.
- **Maintenance:** Consume calories equal to the TDEE.
- **Weight Gain:** Add 250-500 calories to the TDEE, focusing on lean muscle gain to avoid excess fat accumulation.

MEAL TIMING AND FREQUENCY

Importance of Meal Timing and Frequency

For endomorphs, the timing and frequency of meals can influence metabolism, energy levels, and hunger control.

Optimal Meal Timing Strategies

- **Frequent, Smaller Meals:** Consuming smaller, balanced meals every 3-4 hours can help maintain steady blood sugar levels and prevent overeating.
- **Post-Workout Nutrition:** Including a mix of protein and carbohydrates within 30 minutes to an hour after workouts aids in muscle recovery and replenishes glycogen stores.
- **Breakfast:** Starting the day with a high-protein, moderate-carb breakfast can kickstart metabolism and reduce hunger throughout the day.

Sample Meal Schedule

- **Breakfast (7:00 AM):** A mix of proteins and complex carbs, such as scrambled eggs with vegetables and whole-grain toast.
- **Mid-Morning Snack (10:00 AM):** Greek yogurt with a handful of nuts or a protein smoothie.

- **Lunch (1:00 PM):** Grilled chicken salad with mixed greens, quinoa, and an olive oil-based dressing.
- **Afternoon Snack (4:00 PM):** Sliced veggies with hummus or a piece of fruit with nut butter.
- **Dinner (7:00 PM):** Baked salmon with roasted vegetables and a small portion of brown rice.
- **Evening Snack (9:00 PM):** Cottage cheese with berries or a small protein shake.

Additional Tips for Meal Timing

- **Hydration:** Drink plenty of water throughout the day to support metabolism and overall health.
- **Avoid Late-Night Eating:** Minimize food intake close to bedtime to prevent unnecessary calorie storage as fat.

For endomorphs, managing daily caloric intake, maintaining an ideal macronutrient balance, and adhering to a structured meal timing schedule are critical components for achieving and sustaining a healthy weight and optimal body composition.

28-DAY MEAL PLAN

WEEK 1

	BREAKFAST	LUNCH	DINNER	SNACKS
DAY 1	Blueberry Almond Smoothie	Grilled Shrimp Tacos	Spaghetti Squash with Turkey Bolognese	Apple Slices with Almond Butter
DAY 2	Vegetable Omelette	Homemade Mushroom and Barley Soup	Grilled Salmon with Asparagus and Quinoa	Carrot Sticks with Hummus
DAY 3	Keto Breakfast Burrito	Lentil Soup with a Side Salad	Grilled Portobello Mushrooms	Cucumber slices with tzatziki
DAY 4	Greek Yogurt Parfait	Chickpea and Avocado Salad	Endo Guacamole	Air Popped Popcorn
DAY 5	Scrambled Eggs with Spinach and Tomatoes	Chicken and Vegetable Soup	Turkey Meatballs with Zucchini Noodles	Pear Slices
DAY 6	Stuffed Bell Peppers	Tuna Salad in Lettuce Wraps	Grilled Shrimp with Quinoa and Mixed Vegetables	Greek Yogurt with a Drizzle of Honey
DAY 7	Protein Smoothie Recipe	Chickpea and Veggie Salad	Meaty Muffins	Sliced Cucumbers with Guacamole

	BREAKFAST	LUNCH	DINNER	SNACKS
DAY 1	Chia Seed Pudding with Berries	Beef and Broccoli	Herbed Pork Tenderloin	Hard-boiled Egg
DAY 2	Healthy Cauliflower Hash Browns	Lentil and Vegetable Stew	Endo Parmesan Asparagus	Bell Pepper Strips with Hummus
DAY 3	Greek Yogurt with Granola and Blueberries	Quinoa Salad with Roasted Vegetables	Chicken Fajita Bowl	Apple Slices with Peanut Butter
DAY 4	Smoothie Bowl with Kale, Pineapple, and Chia Seeds	Black Bean and Corn Salad	Grilled Salmon with Asparagus and Sweet Potato	Carrot sticks with hummus
DAY 5	Avocado and Egg Breakfast Fowl	Grilled Chicken Salad	Baked Cod with Steamed Carrots and Brown Rice	Pear Slices with Ricotta
DAY 6	Scrambled Eggs with Mushrooms and Spinach	Vegetable Soup with Quinoa	Almond-Crusted Tilapia	Greek Yogurt with Honey
DAY 7	Spinach and Berry Smoothie	Eggplant Parmesan	Baked Chicken Breast with Roasted Brussels Sprouts	Turnip Chips

Repeat Week 1 and Week 2 to complete the 28-Day Meal Plan.
This meal plan includes balanced meals designed to revitalize your metabolism and soothe your digestive system after gallbladder removal. Each week has a mix of lean proteins, complex carbohydrates, healthy fats, and fiber-rich foods to ensure optimal digestive health.

VEGETABLE OMELETTE

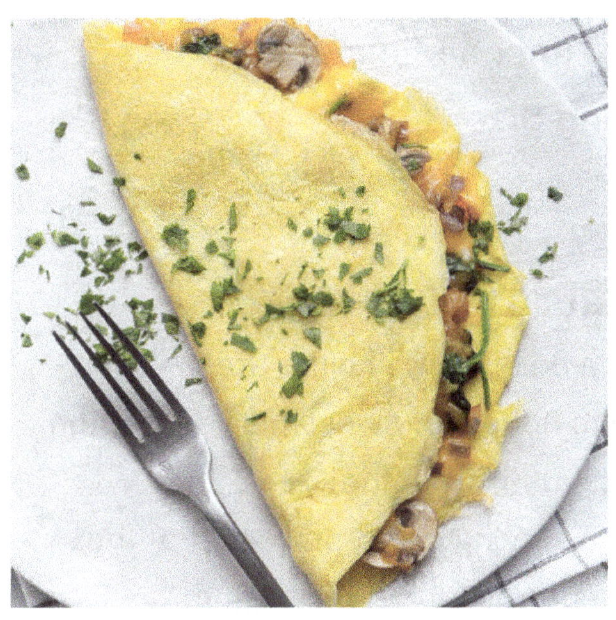

Prep Time: 10 Mins

Serving Size: 1

INGREDIENTS

- 2 whole eggs
- 1 egg white
- 1 cup chopped spinach
- 1/2 cup diced bell peppers
- 1/4 cup diced onions
- 1 tablespoon olive oil
- Salt and pepper to taste

NUTRITIONAL FACTS

- Calories: 300 kcal
- Protein: 20g
- Fats: 20g
- Carbohydrates: 10g

INSTRUCTIONS

- Warm the olive oil in a non-stick skillet over medium heat.
- Sauté the onions and bell peppers until tender.
- Add the spinach and cook until it wilts.
- In a bowl, beat the whole eggs and egg white with salt and pepper.
- Pour the egg mixture over the vegetables in the skillet.
- Cook for 3-4 minutes until the bottom is set.
- Carefully flip the omelette and cook for an additional 2-3 minutes.
- Serve immediately.

GREEK YOGURT PARFAIT

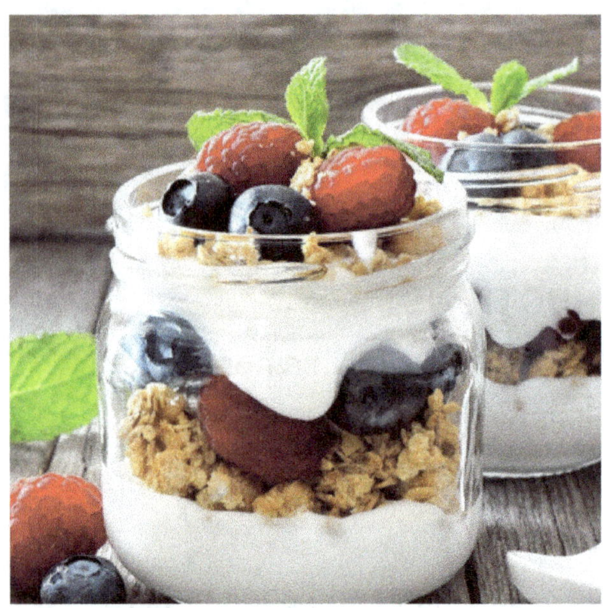

Prep Time: 5 Mins

Serving Size: 1

INSTRUCTIONS

- In a bowl, combine the Greek yogurt with honey (or sweetener) and lemon zest until smooth.
- In a serving glass, place half of the yogurt mixture at the bottom.
- Add a layer of mixed berries on top of the yogurt.
- Sprinkle half of the almonds and chia seeds over the berries.
- Repeat the layers with the remaining yogurt, berries, almonds, and chia seeds.
- Garnish with a few berries and a touch of lemon zest for extra flavor.

INGREDIENTS

- 1 cup plain full-fat Greek yogurt
- 1/4 cup mixed berries (blueberries, raspberries, strawberries)
- 1 tablespoon slivered almonds
- 1 teaspoon chia seeds
- 1 tablespoon honey or a low-calorie sweetener
- A pinch of lemon zest (optional)

NUTRITIONAL FACTS

- Calories: 280 kcal
- Protein: 22g
- Fats: 15g
- Carbohydrates: 18g

AVOCADO AND EGG BREAKFAST BOWL

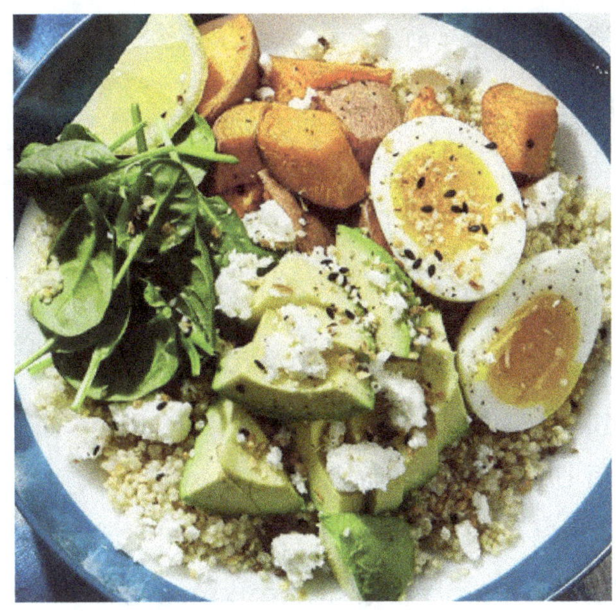

Cook Time: 20 Mins

Serving Size: 1

INGREDIENTS

- 1 ripe avocado
- 2 large eggs
- Salt and pepper to taste
- Optional toppings: cherry tomatoes, green onions, salsa

NUTRITIONAL FACTS

- Calories: 450 kcal
- Protein: 15g
- Fat: 40g
- Carbohydrates: 12g

INSTRUCTIONS

- Preheat your oven to 425°F (220°C).
- Slice the avocado in half and remove the pit. Scoop out a small portion of the avocado flesh to create a bigger cavity.
- Crack one egg into each avocado half.
- Season with salt and pepper.
- Place the avocado halves on a baking sheet and bake in the preheated oven for 15-20 minutes, or until the eggs are cooked to your desired doneness.
- Top with optional ingredients like cherry tomatoes, green onions, or salsa before serving.

PROTEIN SMOOTHIE RECIPE

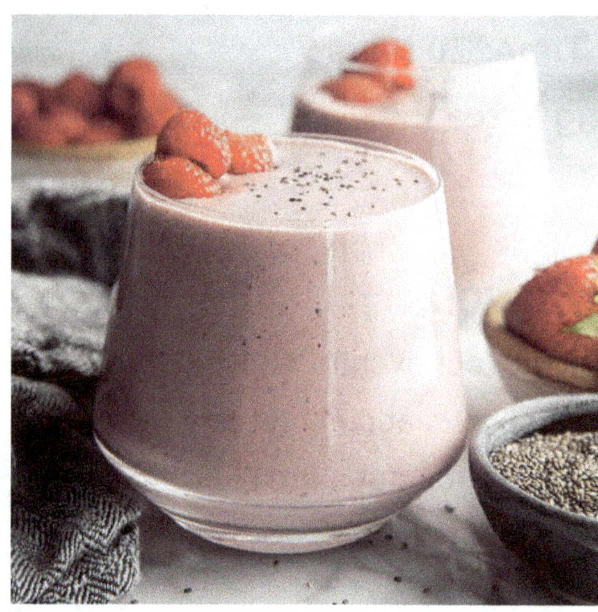

Prep Time: 5 Mins

Serving Size: 1

INSTRUCTIONS

- Combine the protein powder, almond milk, avocado, flaxseeds, and spinach in a blender.
- Add a few ice cubes.
- Blend on high until the mixture is smooth.
- Taste the smoothie and add sweetener if needed, then blend briefly to mix.
- Pour the smoothie into a glass and enjoy immediately.

INGREDIENTS

- 1 scoop whey protein powder (or plant-based protein for a vegan alternative)
- 1 cup unsweetened almond milk
- 1/2 avocado
- 1 tablespoon flaxseeds
- 1/2 cup spinach
- Ice cubes
- Stevia or another low-calorie sweetener to taste

NUTRITIONAL FACTS

- Calories: 350 kcal
- Protein: 25g
- Fat: 22g
- Carbohydrates: 12g

CHIA SEED PUDDING

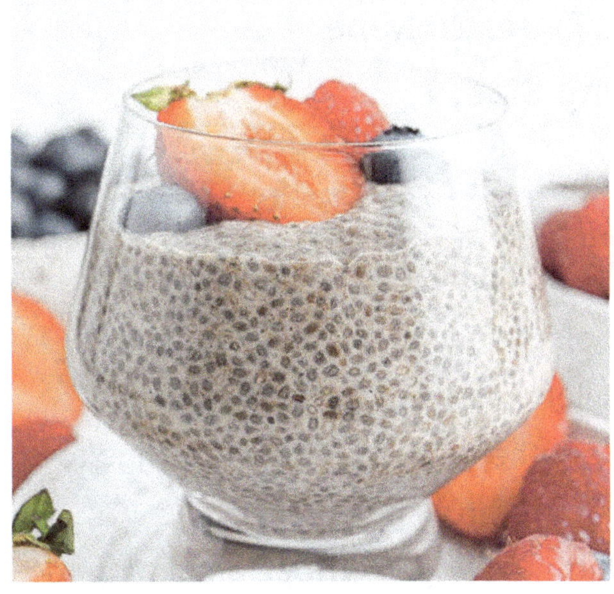

Prep Time: 2 Hrs of soaking

Serving Size: 2

INGREDIENTS

- ⅛ cup (25g) chia seeds
- ¾ cup (150g) unsweetened almond milk
- 1 tablespoon honey (or preferred sweetener)
- ½ teaspoon vanilla extract
- ¼ cup (50g) blueberries
- 1 tablespoon (8g) flaked almonds

INSTRUCTIONS

- In a bowl, combine the chia seeds, almond milk, honey, and vanilla extract.
- Allow the mixture to sit for about one minute, then stir again to break up any clumps.
- Cover the bowl and refrigerate for at least 2 hours, ideally overnight, until the pudding thickens to a creamy consistency.
- Before serving, top with blueberries and flaked almonds for extra flavor and texture.

NUTRITIONAL FACTS

- Calories: 200 kcal
- Carbohydrates: 23g
- Protein: 5g
- Fat: 10g
- Fiber: High (chia seeds are an excellent source of fiber)

KETO BREAKFAST BURRITO

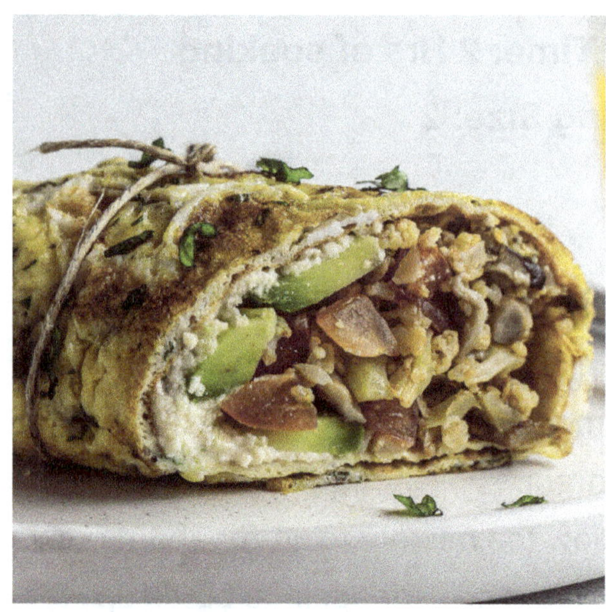

Cook Time: 20 Mins

Serving Size: 2

INGREDIENTS

- 2 Original Egglife Wraps (Zero carbs)
- 2 Breakfast Chicken Sausage Links (Zero carbs)
- 2 strips of Thick Center-Cut Bacon
- 2 Large Eggs
- Optional toppings: Avocado, Cheese, Sour Cream, Sriracha, Zero Carb Cheese Sauce

INSTRUCTIONS

- Cook the bacon and sausage in a skillet until crispy and fully cooked.
- In another pan, scramble the eggs to your preferred consistency.
- Warm the Egglife Wraps according to the package directions to make them flexible.
- Lay out the wraps and evenly distribute the scrambled eggs, bacon, and sausage onto each wrap.
- Add optional ingredients such as avocado or cheese if desired.
- Roll the wraps tightly, tucking in the ends as you roll.

NUTRITIONAL FACTS

- Calories: 300 kcal
- Carbohydrates: 0g net carbs
- Protein: High (exact amount depends on the type of sausage and bacon used)
- Fat: High

STUFFED BELL PEPPERS

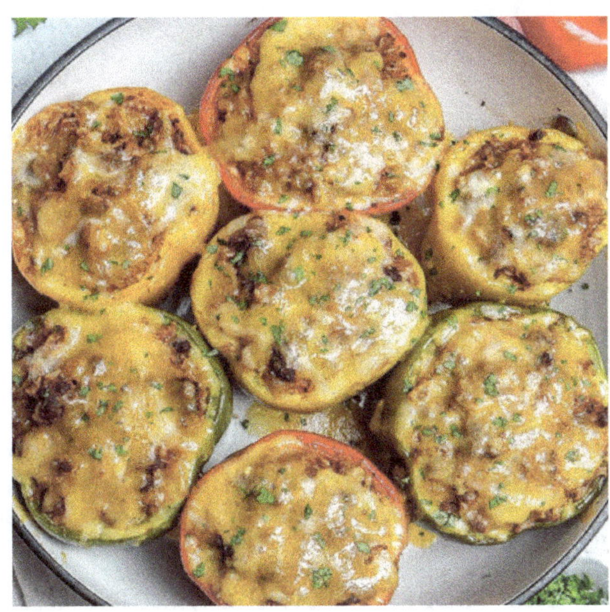

Cook Time: 30 Mins

Serving Size: 4

INGREDIENTS

- 4 large bell peppers (any color)
- 1 lb (450g) lean ground turkey
- 1 cup (150g) cooked quinoa
- 1 cup (240ml) low-sodium tomato sauce
- 1 medium onion, diced
- 2 cloves garlic, minced
- 1 tsp olive oil
- 1 tsp Italian seasoning
- Salt and pepper to taste
- ½ cup (50g) shredded low-fat cheese (optional)

INSTRUCTIONS

- Preheat the oven to 375°F (190°C).
- Cut the tops off the bell peppers and remove the seeds and membranes.
- In a skillet, heat olive oil over medium heat. Add the diced onion and minced garlic, cooking until they become translucent.
- Add the ground turkey to the skillet, cooking until browned. Season with Italian seasoning, salt, and pepper.
- Mix in the cooked quinoa and tomato sauce, cooking for an additional 5 minutes.
- Fill each bell pepper with the turkey mixture and place them in a baking dish.
- Optionally, sprinkle shredded cheese on top of each pepper.
- Bake in the oven for 25-30 minutes, or until the peppers are tender.

NUTRITIONAL FACTS

- Calories: 300 kcal
- Carbohydrates: 20g | Protein: 25g
- Fat: 15g | Fiber: 4g

HEALTHY CAULIFLOWER HASH BROWNS

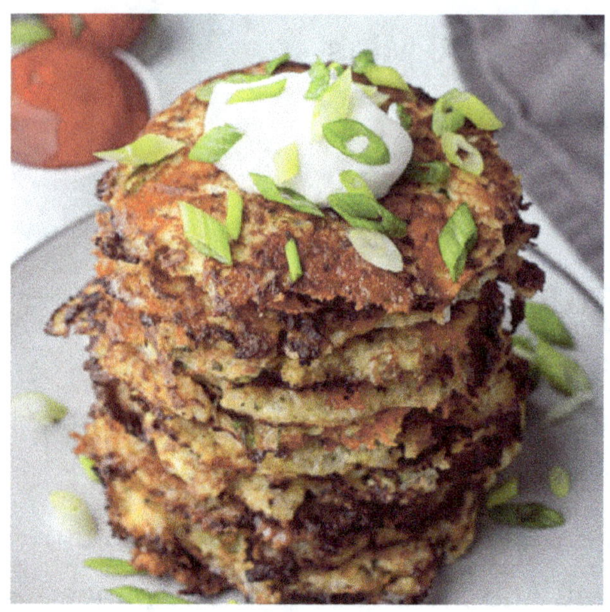

Cook Time: 20 Mins

Serving Size: 6

INGREDIENTS

- 1 lb (450g) cauliflower, grated
- 3 large eggs
- ½ (55g) yellow onion, finely chopped
- 1 tsp salt
- 2 pinches pepper
- 4 oz. (110g) butter or oil (use less if desired)

NUTRITIONAL FACTS

- Calories: 150 kcal
- Carbohydrates: 5g
- Protein: 4g
- Fat: 8-10g (varies with the amount of butter or oil used)
- Fiber: High

INSTRUCTIONS

- Grate the cauliflower using a food processor or grater.
- In a large bowl, combine the grated cauliflower with eggs, chopped onion, salt, and pepper. Allow the mixture to rest for 5–10 minutes.
- Heat a non-stick skillet over medium heat and melt a portion of the butter or oil.
- Scoop portions of the cauliflower mixture into the pan, flattening them to form patties approximately 3–4 inches in diameter.
- Cook for 4–5 minutes on each side until golden brown and crispy.
- Keep the cooked hash browns warm in the oven while preparing the remaining batches.

HOMEMADE MUSHROOM AND BARLEY SOUP

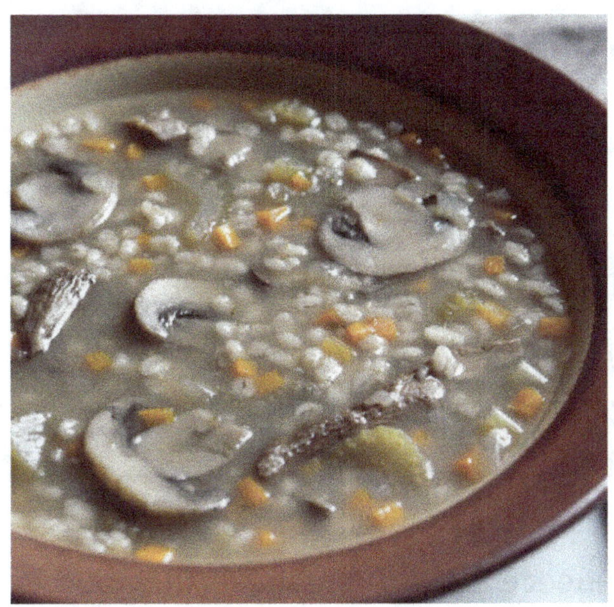

Cook Time: 1 Hour

Serving Size: 8

INGREDIENTS

- 2 tablespoons of olive oil
- 2 tablespoons of unsalted butter
- 1/2 cup of barley, rinsed
- 2 medium-sized onions, finely diced
- 1/2 pound of mushrooms, thinly sliced
- 8 cups of reduced sodium chicken broth
- 1 large carrot, thinly sliced
- 1/2 teaspoon of salt
- 1/4 teaspoon of ground black pepper
- 2 tablespoons of minced parsley or dill (for garnish)
- Sour cream (optional, for serving)

INSTRUCTIONS

- Begin by dicing the onions, slicing the mushrooms, and thinly slicing the carrot.
- In a large soup pot, heat the olive oil and butter over medium heat.
- Add the rinsed barley and diced onions, cooking for approximately 5 minutes while stirring frequently.
- Incorporate the sliced mushrooms into the pot and cook for an additional 5 minutes or until the mushroom liquid has evaporated.
- Pour in the reduced sodium chicken broth, add the sliced carrot, salt, and pepper. Bring the soup to a boil, then reduce the heat to a simmer.
- Cover the pot and let it simmer on low heat for about 1 hour, remembering to stir every 15 minutes.
- Just before serving, sprinkle the soup with minced parsley or dill.
- Enjoy your flavorful homemade mushroom and barley soup!

TUNA SALAD IN LETTUCE WRAPS

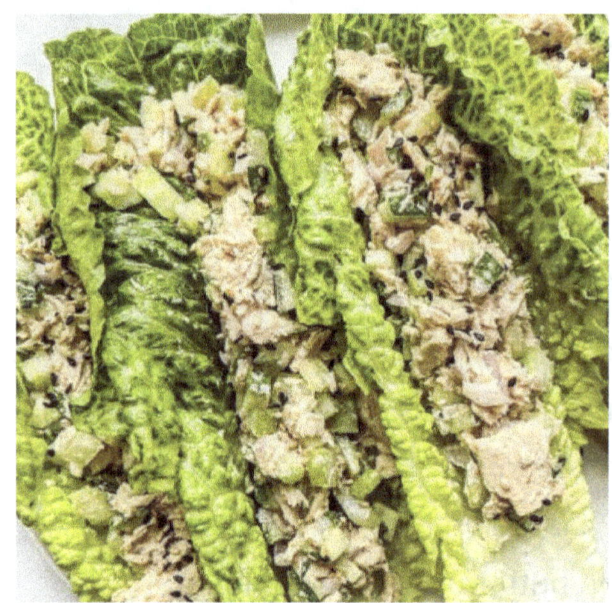

Prep Time: 10 Mins

Serving Size: 2

INSTRUCTIONS

- In a large bowl, mix the drained tuna with the low-fat mayonnaise or Greek yogurt, celery, red onion, capers, mustard, and parsley.
- Squeeze in the lemon juice, then add salt and pepper to taste. Stir everything together until well mixed.
- Rinse and pat dry the lettuce leaves. Place a portion of the tuna mixture into the center of each leaf.
- Serve immediately for a light, protein-rich meal.

INGREDIENTS

- 2 cans (12 oz each) of tuna in water, drained
- 1/4 cup low-fat mayonnaise or Greek yogurt
- 1/4 cup finely chopped celery
- 2 tablespoons minced red onion
- 1 tablespoon capers, rinsed and chopped
- 1 tablespoon whole grain mustard
- 2 tablespoons chopped fresh parsley
- Juice of 1 lemon
- Salt and pepper to taste
- 8 large lettuce leaves (such as Romaine or Butter lettuce)

NUTRITIONAL FACTS

- Calories: 150kcal
- Protein: 25g
- Carbohydrates: 5g
- Fat: 5g
- Fiber: 1g
- Sugars: 2g

BEEF AND BROCCOLI STIR-FRY

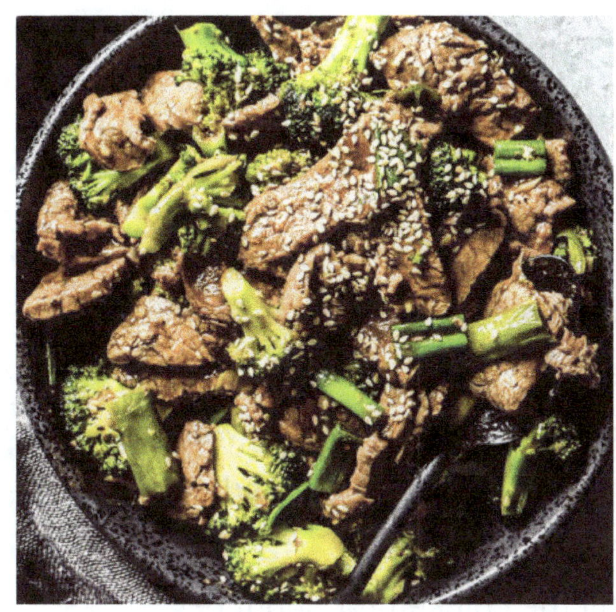

Cook Time: 20 Mins
Serving Size: 4

INGREDIENTS

- 1 lb beef sirloin, thinly sliced
- 3 cups broccoli florets
- 2 Tbsp olive oil
- 1 Tbsp minced garlic
- 1/2 cup low-sodium beef broth
- 2 Tbsp low-sodium soy sauce
- 1 Tbsp oyster sauce
- 1 tsp cornstarch
- 1 tsp sesame oil
- Salt and pepper to taste

NUTRITIONAL FACTS

- Calories: 260kcal | Protein: 24g
- Carbohydrates: 10g | Fiber: 3g
- Sugars: 2g
- Fat: 13g

INSTRUCTIONS

- In a small bowl, combine the beef broth, soy sauce, oyster sauce, cornstarch, and sesame oil. Whisk until well blended and set aside.
- Heat the olive oil in a large skillet over medium-high heat. Add the minced garlic and sauté for about 30 seconds until fragrant.
- Add the thinly sliced beef to the skillet and stir-fry until browned, then remove from the skillet and set aside.
- In the same skillet, add the broccoli florets and stir-fry until they are bright green and tender-crisp.
- Return the cooked beef to the skillet with the broccoli.
- Pour the sauce mixture over the beef and broccoli, stirring well to coat everything evenly. Cook for an additional 2-3 minutes until the sauce thickens.
- Season with salt and pepper to taste before serving.

GRILLED CHICKEN SALAD

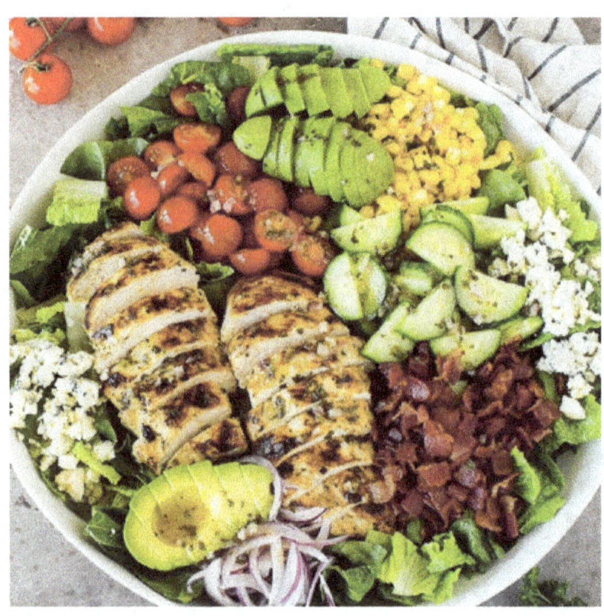

Cook Time: 20 Mins

Serving Size: 4

INGREDIENTS

- 4 boneless, skinless chicken breasts
- 1 tablespoon olive oil
- 1 teaspoon garlic powder
- Salt and pepper to taste
- 8 cups mixed greens (lettuce, spinach, arugula)
- 1 cup cherry tomatoes, halved
- 1 cucumber, sliced
- 1/4 red onion, thinly sliced
- 1/2 avocado, sliced
- 1/4 cup crumbled feta cheese
- 2 tablespoons balsamic vinegar
- 1 tablespoon Dijon mustard
- 1 tablespoon honey
- 3 tablespoons extra virgin olive oil

INSTRUCTIONS

- Preheat your grill to medium-high heat.
- Coat the chicken breasts with olive oil and season them with garlic powder, salt, and pepper.
- Grill the chicken for about 6-7 minutes on each side, or until the internal temperature reaches 165°F.
- Allow the chicken to rest for a few minutes before slicing it.
- In a large bowl, mix the greens, cherry tomatoes, cucumber, and red onion.
- In a separate small bowl, whisk together the balsamic vinegar, Dijon mustard, honey, and extra virgin olive oil to make the dressing.
- Toss the salad with the dressing.
- Top the salad with the sliced chicken, avocado, and crumbled feta cheese.

NUTRITIONAL FACTS

- Calories: 380kcal | Protein: 32g
- Carbohydrates: 14g | Fat: 22g
- Fiber: 5g | Sugars: 7g

EGGPLANT PARMESAN

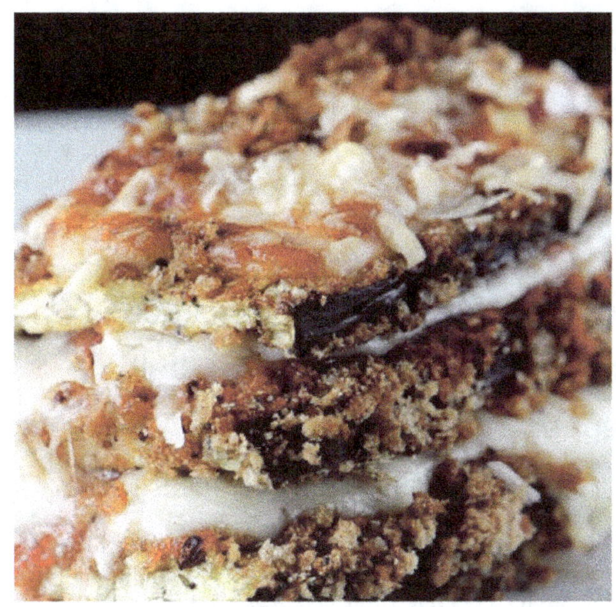

Cook Time: 60 Mins

Serving Size: 6

INSTRUCTIONS

- Preheat oven to 475°F (240°C).
- Slice eggplants into 1/2-inch rounds.
- Whisk egg whites with water until frothy. Dip eggplant slices into the mixture, then coat with Parmesan.
- Place slices on a parchment-lined baking sheet, sprinkle with garlic powder, and spray with olive oil. Bake for 20 minutes, flip, and bake for 10 more minutes.
- Lower oven to 350°F (180°C).
- In a baking dish, layer tomato puree, crushed tomatoes, eggplant, mozzarella, and basil. Repeat until all ingredients are used.
- Bake for 25-30 minutes until cheese is melted and bubbly.

INGREDIENTS

- 2 large eggplants (about 2 pounds)
- 2 cups low-sodium tomato puree
- 1 cup crushed tomatoes
- 1/2 cup chopped fresh basil leaves
- 1 cup part-skim shredded mozzarella cheese
- 1/2 cup reduced-fat grated Parmesan cheese
- 2 egg whites
- 2 tablespoons water
- Garlic powder, to taste
- Salt and pepper, to taste
- Olive oil spray

NUTRITIONAL FACTS

- Calories: 250kcal
- Carbohydrates: 20g
- Protein: 15g
- Fat: 10g
- Fiber: 6g

CHICKPEA AND VEGGIE SALAD

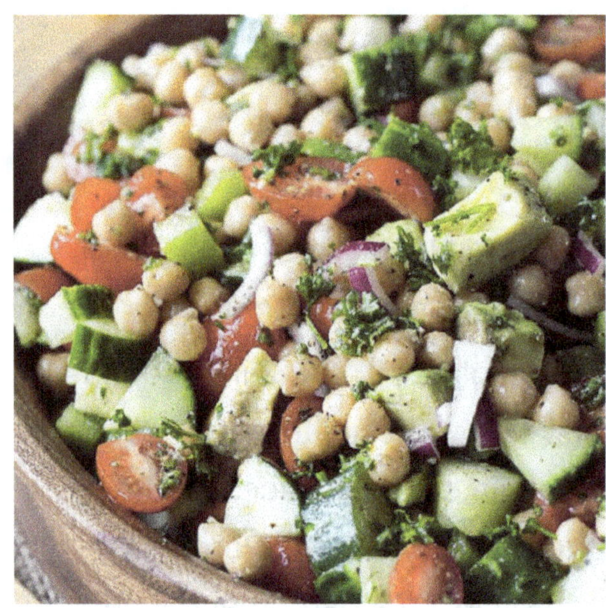

Prep Time: 15 Mins

Serving Size: 4

INSTRUCTIONS

- In a large bowl, mix the chickpeas, cherry tomatoes, cucumber, bell pepper, and red onion.
- In a small bowl, whisk together the olive oil, lemon juice, smoked paprika, salt, and pepper to make the dressing.
- Pour the dressing over the chickpea and vegetable mixture and toss to ensure everything is evenly coated.
- Garnish with fresh parsley before serving.

INGREDIENTS

- 1 can (15 oz) chickpeas, drained and rinsed
- 1 cup cherry tomatoes, halved
- 1 medium cucumber, diced
- 1 red bell pepper, diced
- 1/2 red onion, thinly sliced
- 1/4 cup fresh parsley, chopped
- 2 tablespoons olive oil
- 1 tablespoon lemon juice
- 1 teaspoon smoked paprika
- Salt and pepper to taste

NUTRITIONAL FACTS

- Calories: 180kcal
- Carbohydrates: 20g
- Protein: 6g
- Fat: 8g
- Fiber: 5g

GRILLED SHRIMP TACOS

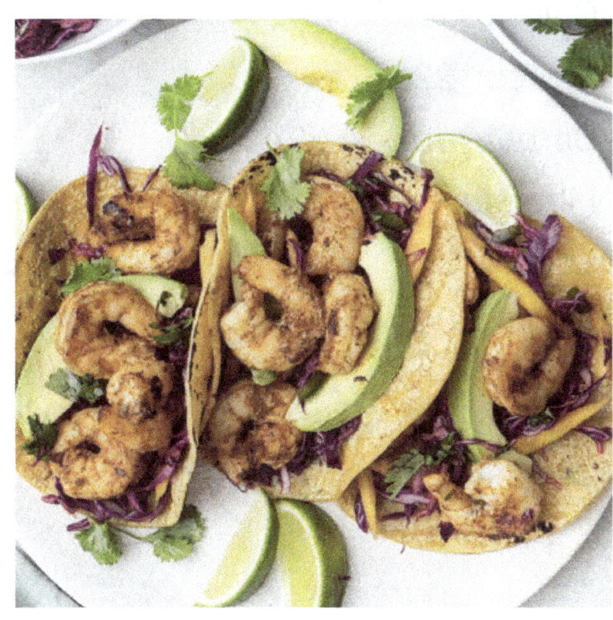

Prep Time: 40 Mins

Serving Size: 2

INSTRUCTIONS

- Mix olive oil, garlic, chili powder, cumin, smoked paprika, salt, pepper, and lime juice in a bowl.
- Add shrimp, toss to coat, and marinate for 15 minutes.
- Preheat grill to medium-high.
- Thread shrimp onto skewers.
- Grill shrimp 2-3 minutes per side until pink and opaque.
- Mix Greek yogurt, lime juice, cilantro, salt, and pepper in a small bowl.
- Warm tortillas on the grill or in a skillet.
- Place grilled shrimp on tortillas.
- Top with cabbage, avocado, cilantro, red onion, and jalapeño (if using).
- Drizzle with sauce and serve with lime wedges.

INGREDIENTS

For the Shrimp:

- 1 lb large shrimp, peeled and deveined
- 2 tbsp olive oil
- 2 cloves garlic, minced
- 1 tsp chili powder
- 1 tsp cumin
- 1 tsp smoked paprika
- 1/2 tsp salt
- 1/4 tsp black pepper
- Juice of 1 lime

For the Tacos:

- 8 small corn tortillas
- 1 cup shredded red cabbage
- 1 avocado, sliced
- 1/2 cup chopped cilantro
- 1/4 cup diced red onion

INGREDIENTS

- 1 jalapeño, thinly sliced (optional)
- 1 lime, cut into wedges

For the Sauce:

- 1/4 cup Greek yogurt
- 1 tbsp lime juice
- 1 tbsp finely chopped cilantro
- Salt and pepper to taste

NUTRITIONAL FACTS

- Calories: 300kcal
- Protein: 22g
- Carbohydrates: 22g
- Fiber: 6g
- Sugars: 3g
- Fat: 15g

SPAGHETTI SQUASH WITH TURKEY BOLOGNESE

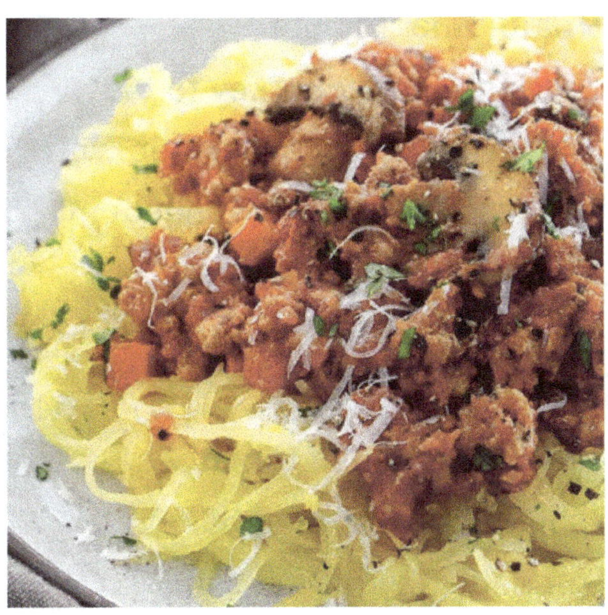

Prep Time: 1 Hour

Serving Size: 4

INSTRUCTIONS

Preparing the Spaghetti Squash:

- Preheat the oven to 400°F (200°C).
- Cut the spaghetti squash in half lengthwise and scoop out the seeds.
- Brush the inside of each half with olive oil and season with salt and pepper.
- Place the squash halves cut side down on a baking sheet lined with parchment paper.
- Roast in the preheated oven for 35-40 minutes, until the squash is tender and easily pierced with a fork.
- Once done, let it cool slightly. Use a fork to scrape out the strands of squash into a bowl. Set aside.

Preparing the Turkey Bolognese:

- Heat the olive oil in a large skillet over medium heat.
- Add the chopped onion, carrot, celery, and bell pepper. Cook until the vegetables are soft, about 5-7 minutes.

INGREDIENTS

For the Spaghetti Squash:

- 1 medium spaghetti squash
- 1 tablespoon olive oil
- Salt and pepper to taste

For the Turkey Bolognese:

- 1 pound ground turkey (preferably lean, 93% lean)
- 1 medium onion, finely chopped
- 2 cloves garlic, minced
- 1 large carrot, finely diced
- 1 celery stalk, finely diced
- 1 red bell pepper, finely diced
- 1 can (28 ounces) crushed tomatoes (no added sugar)
- 1 tablespoon tomato paste
- 1/2 cup chicken broth (low sodium)

INGREDIENTS

- 1 teaspoon dried basil
- 1 teaspoon dried oregano
- 1/2 teaspoon dried thyme
- Salt and pepper to taste
- 1 tablespoon olive oil
- Fresh parsley, chopped (optional, for garnish)

NUTRITIONAL FACTS

- Calories: 320 kcal
- Protein: 30g
- Fat: 14g
- Carbohydrates: 20g
- Fiber: 5g
- Sugars: 10g

INSTRUCTIONS

- Add the minced garlic and cook for another minute.
- Add the ground turkey to the skillet. Cook, breaking it up with a spoon, until it's no longer pink, about 8-10 minutes.
- Stir in the tomato paste and cook for 1-2 minutes.
- Add the crushed tomatoes, chicken broth, dried basil, oregano, thyme, salt, and pepper. Stir well to combine.
- Bring the mixture to a boil, then reduce the heat and let it simmer uncovered for 20-25 minutes, until the sauce has thickened.
- Taste and adjust seasoning if necessary.

Assembling the Dish:

- Divide the spaghetti squash strands among four plates.
- Top each plate with a generous portion of turkey bolognese sauce.
- Garnish with fresh parsley if desired.

GRILLED PORTOBELLO MUSHROOMS

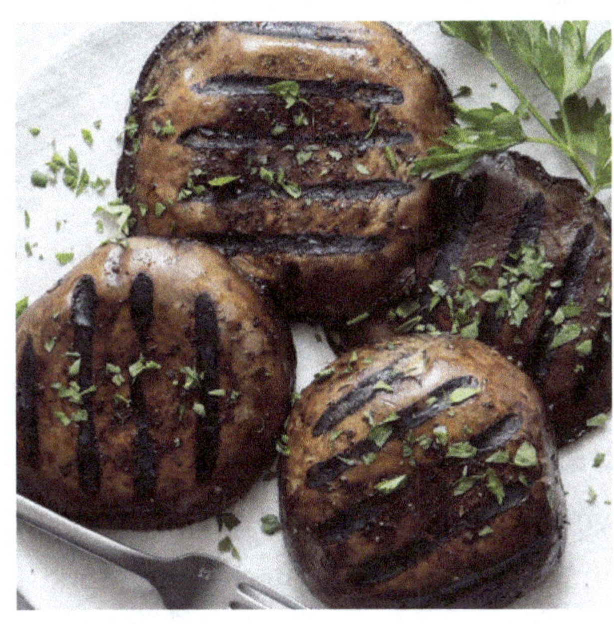

INGREDIENTS

- 4 large Portobello mushrooms, stems removed
- 2 tablespoons olive oil
- 2 tablespoons balsamic vinegar
- 2 cloves garlic, minced
- 1 teaspoon dried thyme
- 1 teaspoon dried rosemary
- Salt and pepper to taste
- Fresh parsley, chopped (optional, for garnish)

NUTRITIONAL FACTS

- Calories: 90kcal | Protein: 3g
- Carbohydrates: 7g
- Dietary Fiber: 2g
- Sugars: 3g
- Fat: 7g

Prep Time: 20 Mins
Grilling Time: 14 Mins
Serving Size: 1

INSTRUCTIONS

- Clean the Portobello mushrooms by wiping them with a damp cloth. Remove the stems and set them aside.
- In a small bowl, mix together the olive oil, balsamic vinegar, minced garlic, thyme, rosemary, salt, and pepper.
- Brush the marinade generously over both sides of the mushrooms. Let them sit for about 15-20 minutes to absorb the flavors.
- reheat your grill to medium-high heat (about 375°F to 400°F or 190°C to 204°C).
- Place the mushrooms on the grill, gill side up, and cook for about 5-7 minutes.
- Flip the mushrooms and cook for another 5-7 minutes, until they are tender and have nice grill marks.
- Remove the mushrooms from the grill and let them rest for a couple of minutes.
- Slice the mushrooms if desired, and garnish with fresh parsley.

HERBED PORK TENDERLOIN

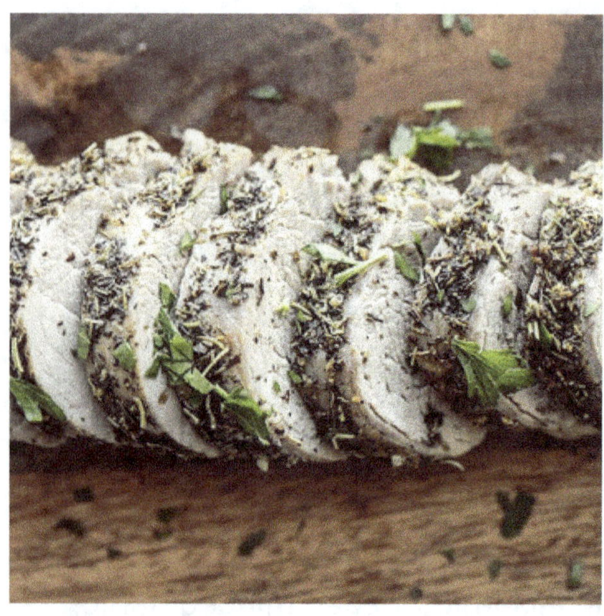

Cook Time: 35 Mins

Serving Size: 4

INGREDIENTS

- 2 pork tenderloins (about 1 pound each)
- 2 tablespoons olive oil
- 2 cloves garlic, minced
- 1 tablespoon fresh rosemary, chopped
- 1 tablespoon fresh thyme leaves
- 1 tablespoon fresh parsley, chopped
- Salt and pepper to taste

INSTRUCTIONS

- Preheat your oven to 375°F (190°C).
- In a small bowl, mix together the olive oil, minced garlic, chopped rosemary, thyme, parsley, salt, and pepper.
- Rub the herb mixture all over the pork tenderloins, ensuring they are evenly coated.
- Heat a skillet over medium-high heat. Once hot, sear the pork tenderloins on all sides until browned, about 2-3 minutes per side.
- Transfer the pork tenderloins to a baking dish and roast in the preheated oven for 20-25 minutes or until the internal temperature reaches 145°F (63°C) for medium-rare or 160°F (71°C) for medium.
- Once cooked, remove the pork tenderloins from the oven and let them rest for 5 minutes before slicing.
- Serve the sliced pork tenderloin with your favorite side dishes.

NUTRITIONAL FACTS

- Calories: 250 kcal
- Protein: 25g
- Fat: 14g
- Carbohydrates: 2g
- Fiber: 1g

CHICKEN FAJITA BOWL

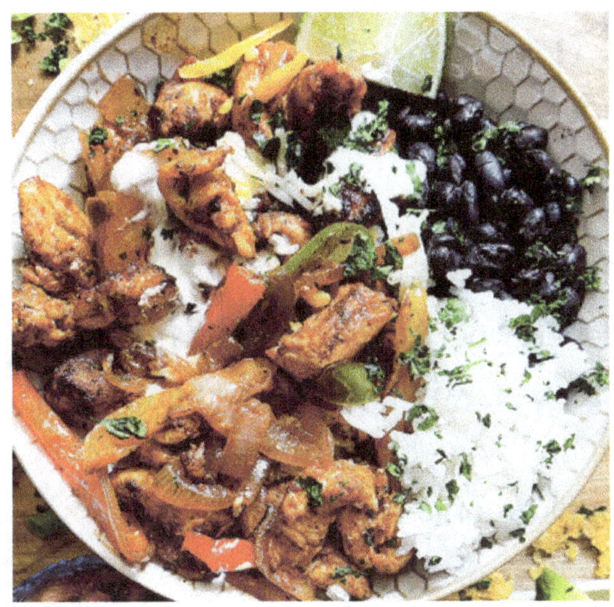

Cook Time: 30 Mins

Serving Size: 2

INSTRUCTIONS

- In a bowl, combine the sliced chicken with chili powder, cumin, paprika, salt, pepper, and 1 tablespoon of olive oil. Mix well to coat the chicken evenly. Let it marinate for at least 30 minutes in the refrigerator.

- Heat the remaining tablespoon of olive oil in a skillet over medium-high heat. Add the marinated chicken strips and cook until they are browned and cooked through, about 5-6 minutes per side. Remove from the skillet and set aside.

- In the same skillet, add the sliced bell peppers and onions. Cook until they are tender and slightly charred, about 5-7 minutes.

- Divide the cooked rice or quinoa among serving bowls. Top with the cooked chicken, sautéed vegetables, and sliced avocado. Add any optional toppings as desired.

INGREDIENTS

- 2 boneless, skinless chicken breasts, sliced into strips
- 2 bell peppers (red, green, or yellow), sliced
- 1 onion, sliced
- 2 tablespoons olive oil
- 2 teaspoons chili powder
- 1 teaspoon cumin
- 1 teaspoon paprika
- Salt and pepper to taste
- 2 cups cooked brown rice or quinoa
- 1 avocado, sliced
- Optional toppings: salsa, Greek yogurt (as a substitute for sour cream), lime wedges, chopped cilantro

ALMOND-CRUSTED TILAPIA

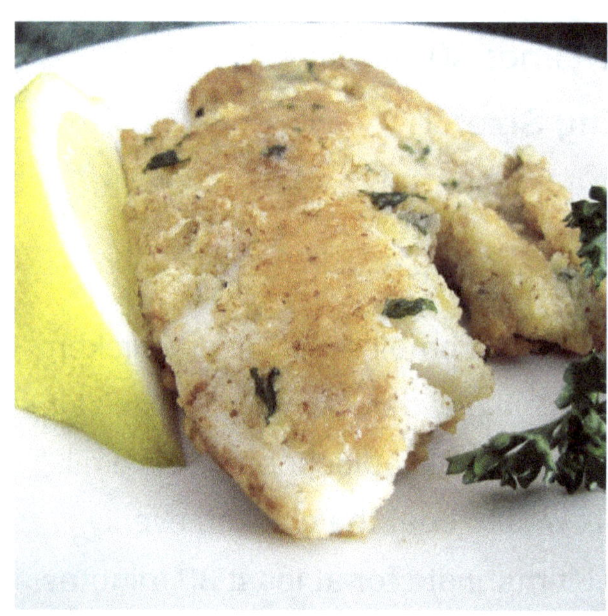

Cook Time: 25 Mins

Serving Size: 4

INSTRUCTIONS

- Preheat your oven to 375°F (190°C).
- In a shallow dish, mix together the almond flour, chopped almonds, paprika, garlic powder, salt, and pepper.
- Dip each tilapia fillet into the beaten eggs, then coat it with the almond mixture, pressing gently to adhere.
- In a large skillet, heat olive oil over medium-high heat. Once hot, add the coated tilapia fillets and cook for 2-3 minutes on each side until golden brown.
- Transfer the skillet to the preheated oven and bake for an additional 10-12 minutes, or until the tilapia is cooked through and flakes easily with a fork.
- Once cooked, serve the almond-crusted tilapia hot, garnished with fresh herbs if desired.

INGREDIENTS

- 4 tilapia fillets
- 1 cup almond flour
- 1/2 cup finely chopped almonds
- 1 teaspoon paprika
- 1 teaspoon garlic powder
- Salt and pepper to taste
- 2 eggs, beaten
- Olive oil for frying

NUTRITIONAL FACTS

- Calories: 350 kcal
- Protein: 30g
- Fat: 20g
- Carbohydrates: 10g
- Fiber: 4g

MEATY MUFFINS

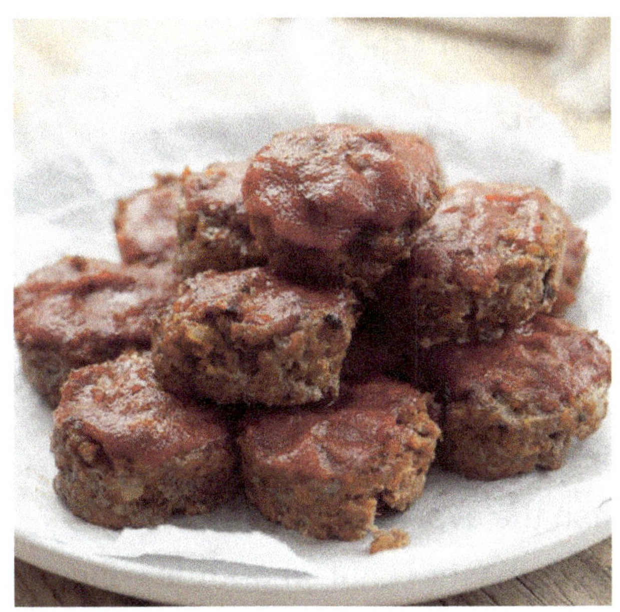

Cook Time: 30 Mins

Serving Size: 12

INGREDIENTS

- 500g lean ground beef
- 1 onion, finely chopped
- 2 cloves garlic, minced
- 1 cup rolled oats
- 1/2 cup grated zucchini
- 1/2 cup grated carrot
- 1/4 cup chopped parsley
- 2 eggs
- 1/4 cup low-fat milk
- Salt and pepper to taste
- Cooking spray or olive oil for greasing

NUTRITIONAL FACTS

- Calories: 180 kcal | Protein: 15g
- Carbohydrates: 10g | Fat: 8g
- Fiber: 2g

INSTRUCTIONS

- Preheat your oven to 180°C (350°F).
- In a large mixing bowl, combine the lean ground beef, chopped onion, minced garlic, rolled oats, grated zucchini, grated carrot, chopped parsley, eggs, and milk.
- Season the mixture with salt and pepper according to your taste preferences.
- Mix all the ingredients thoroughly until well combined.
- Lightly grease a muffin tin with cooking spray or olive oil.
- Spoon the meat mixture evenly into the muffin tin, filling each cup about 3/4 full.
- Place the muffin tin in the preheated oven and bake for 25-30 minutes, or until the meat muffins are cooked through and golden brown on top.
- Once cooked, remove the muffin tin from the oven and let the meaty muffins cool for a few minutes before serving.

ENDO GUACAMOLE

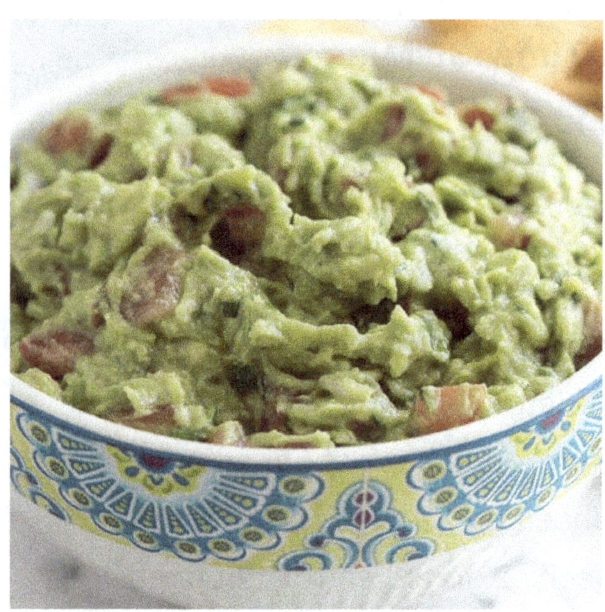

Prep Time: 10 Mins

Serving Size: 4

INSTRUCTIONS

- Cut the avocados in half, remove the pits, and scoop the flesh into a mixing bowl.
- Mash the avocados with a fork or potato masher until smooth, leaving some chunks if desired.
- Add the diced onion, tomato, jalapeño (if using), minced garlic, and chopped cilantro to the bowl.
- Squeeze the lime juice over the mixture and season with salt and pepper.
- Gently stir until all ingredients are well combined.
- Taste and adjust seasoning if necessary.
- Serve immediately with your choice of veggies or whole grain chips.

INGREDIENTS

- 2 ripe avocados
- 1 small onion, finely diced
- 1 ripe tomato, diced
- 1 jalapeño pepper, seeded and minced (optional, adjust to taste)
- 1 lime, juiced
- 2 cloves garlic, minced
- 1/4 cup chopped fresh cilantro
- Salt and pepper to taste

NUTRITIONAL FACTS

- Calories: 160 kcal | Fat: 14g
- Carbohydrates: 10g
- Dietary Fiber: 7g
- Sugars: 2g
- Protein: 2g

ENDO PARMESAN ASPARAGUS

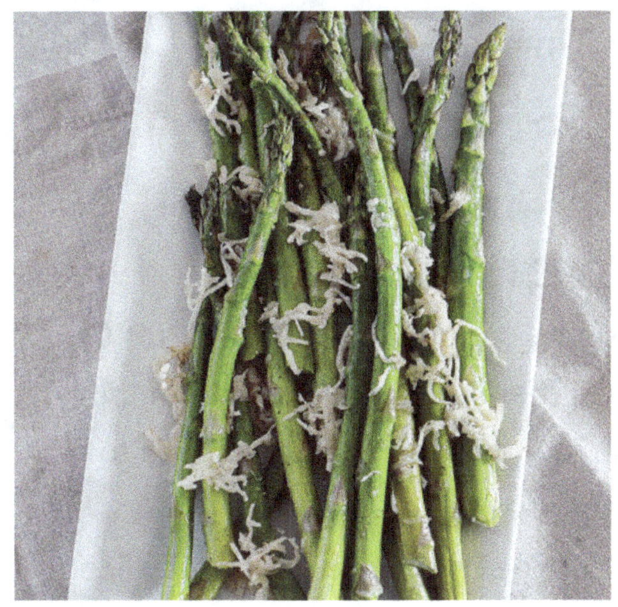

Cook Time: 15 Mins

Serving Size: 4

INGREDIENTS

- 1 bunch of fresh asparagus spears
- 1/4 cup grated Parmesan cheese
- 2 tablespoons olive oil
- 2 cloves garlic, minced
- Salt and black pepper to taste
- Optional: lemon wedges for serving

NUTRITIONAL FACTS

- Calories: 120 kcal
- Total Fat: 9g
- Total Carbohydrates: 6g
- Dietary Fiber: 3g
- Sugars: 2g
- Protein: 5g

INSTRUCTIONS

- Preheat your oven to 400°F (200°C).
- Wash the asparagus spears and trim off the tough ends.
- In a small bowl, mix together the olive oil, minced garlic, salt, and black pepper.
- Arrange the asparagus spears in a single layer on a baking sheet.
- Drizzle the olive oil mixture over the asparagus, making sure they are evenly coated.
- Sprinkle the grated Parmesan cheese over the asparagus.
- Bake in the preheated oven for 12-15 minutes, or until the asparagus is tender and the cheese is golden brown.
- Serve hot, optionally with lemon wedges on the side.

TURNIP CHIPS

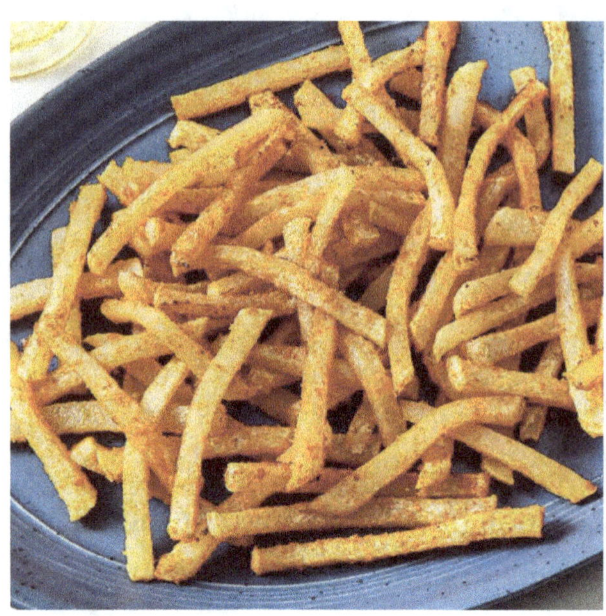

Cook Time: 20 Mins

Serving Size: 4

INGREDIENTS

- 2 large turnips
- 1 tablespoon olive oil
- Salt and pepper to taste
- Optional: herbs or spices of your choice (such as paprika, garlic powder, or rosemary)

NUTRITIONAL FACTS

- Calories: 60 kcal
- Total Fat: 3.5g
- Total Carbohydrates: 7g
- Dietary Fiber: 2g
- Sugars: 3g
- Protein: 1g

INSTRUCTIONS

- Preheat your oven to 400°F (200°C).
- Peel the turnips and slice them thinly, aiming for consistent thickness to ensure even cooking.
- In a large bowl, toss the turnip slices with olive oil until they are evenly coated.
- Season with salt, pepper, and any additional herbs or spices you prefer.
- Arrange the turnip slices in a single layer on a baking sheet lined with parchment paper.
- Bake in the preheated oven for 15-20 minutes, or until the chips are golden brown and crispy, flipping them halfway through the cooking time for even browning.
- Once done, remove from the oven and let them cool slightly before serving.

PEAR SLICES WITH RICOTTA

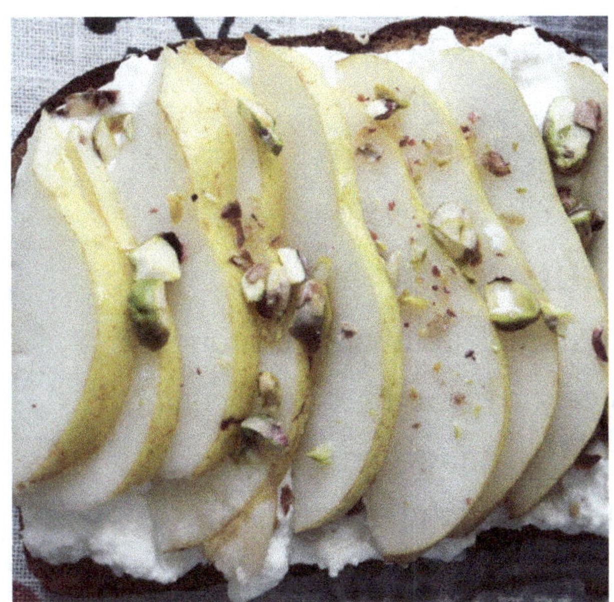

Cook Time: 10 Mins

Serving Size: 4

INGREDIENTS

- 2 medium pears, ripe but firm
- 1 cup ricotta cheese (preferably low-fat)
- 1 tablespoon honey or agave syrup (optional)
- 1/2 teaspoon vanilla extract
- 1/4 teaspoon ground cinnamon
- 1/4 cup chopped walnuts or almonds (optional)
- Fresh mint leaves for garnish (optional)

NUTRITIONAL FACTS

- Calories: 150kcal | Protein: 6g
- Carbohydrates: 22g
- Dietary Fiber: 4g
- Sugars: 16g | Fat: 5g

INSTRUCTIONS

- Wash the pears thoroughly.
- Cut each pear in half lengthwise and remove the core using a melon baller or small spoon.
- Slice each half into thin, even slices.
- In a medium bowl, combine the ricotta cheese, honey (if using), and vanilla extract.
- Stir until the mixture is smooth and well combined.
- Arrange the pear slices on a serving platter.
- Spoon a dollop of the ricotta mixture onto each pear slice.
- Sprinkle ground cinnamon over the top.
- If desired, add a sprinkle of chopped nuts for extra crunch and garnish with fresh mint leaves.
- Serve immediately or chill in the refrigerator for 10-15 minutes before serving for a refreshing treat.

CUCUMBER SLICES WITH TZATZIKI

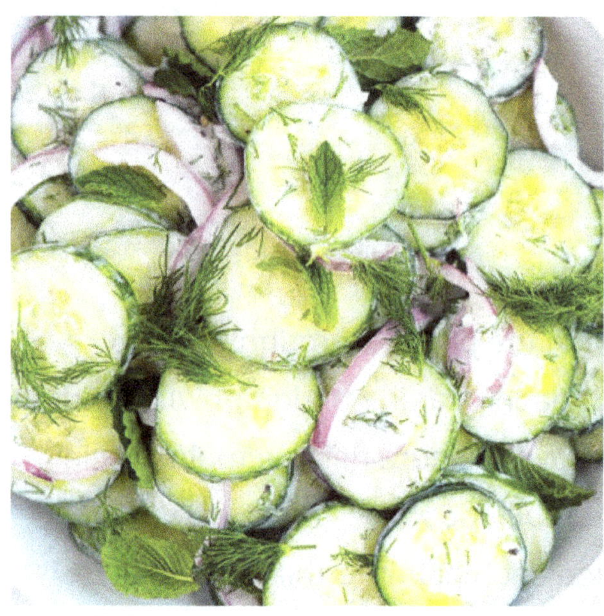

Cook Time: 30 Mins

Serving Size: 4

INSTRUCTIONS

- Wash the cucumbers thoroughly.
- Slice the cucumbers thinly using a knife or mandoline.
- Optional: Lightly sprinkle the cucumber slices with sea salt and set aside for 10 minutes to draw out excess moisture. Pat dry with a paper towel.
- Grate the cucumber and squeeze out the excess water using a cheesecloth or paper towels.
- In a medium bowl, combine the Greek yogurt, grated cucumber, minced garlic, lemon juice, olive oil, dill, sea salt, and black pepper.
- Mix well until all ingredients are fully incorporated.
- Cover and refrigerate the tzatziki for at least 30 minutes to allow the flavors to meld together.
- Arrange the cucumber slices on a serving platter.
- Serve the cucumber slices with a side of tzatziki for dipping.

INGREDIENTS

For the Cucumber Slices:

- 2 large cucumbers, sliced thinly
- 1/4 teaspoon sea salt (optional)

For the Tzatziki:

- 1 cup Greek yogurt (full-fat or 2%)
- 1 medium cucumber, grated and excess water squeezed out
- 2 cloves garlic, minced
- 1 tablespoon fresh lemon juice
- 1 tablespoon extra virgin olive oil
- 1 tablespoon fresh dill, chopped (or 1 teaspoon dried dill)
- 1/2 teaspoon sea salt
- 1/4 teaspoon black pepper

HARD BOILED EGGS

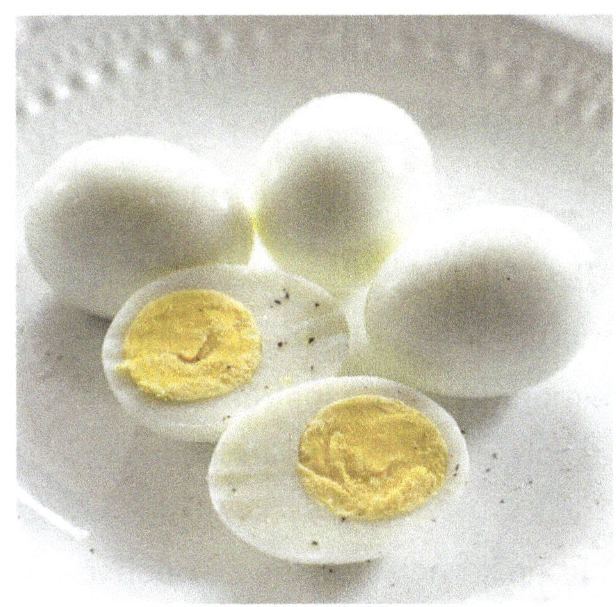

Cook Time: 12 Mins

Serving Size: 2

INSTRUCTIONS

- Prepare: Place eggs in a pot, cover with water.
- Boil: Bring to a rolling boil over high heat.
- Cook: Cover pot, remove from heat, let sit for 9-12 minutes.
- Cool: Transfer eggs to an ice bath for 5 minutes.
- Peel and Serve: Peel under running water.

INGREDIENTS

- 4 large eggs
- Water (enough to cover the eggs in the pot)
- Ice cubes (for the ice bath)

NUTRITIONAL FACTS

- Calories: 140kcal
- Protein: 12g
- Fat: 10g
- Saturated Fat: 3g
- Carbohydrates: 1g
- Fiber: 0g
- Sugars: 0g

AIR POPPED POPCORN

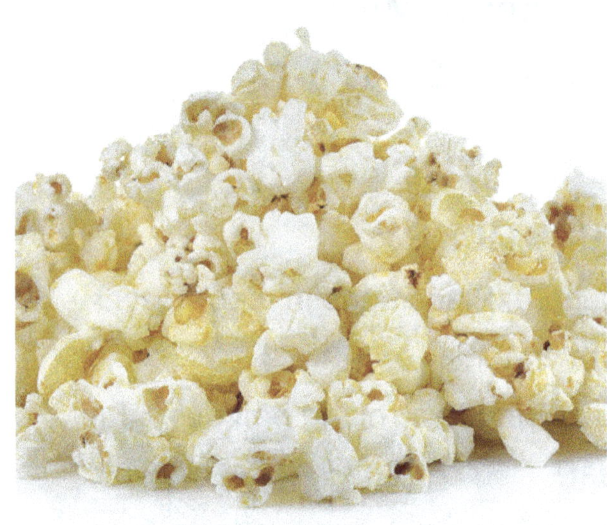

Popping Time: 5 Mins

Serving Size: 3

INSTRUCTIONS

- Set up your air popper according to the manufacturer's instructions.
- Measure out 1/4 cup of popcorn kernels.
- Pour the kernels into the air popper and turn it on. Place a large bowl under the chute to catch the popped popcorn.
- Once the popping slows down to about 2-3 seconds between pops, turn off the popper.
- Lightly spray the popcorn with olive oil if you desire a bit of added flavor and to help seasonings stick.
- Sprinkle sea salt and nutritional yeast over the popcorn. Toss well to evenly distribute the seasoning.

INGREDIENTS

- 1/4 cup popcorn kernels
- 1/4 teaspoon sea salt (optional)
- 1 teaspoon nutritional yeast (optional, for a cheesy flavor)
- Olive oil spray (optional, for light coating)

NUTRITIONAL FACTS

- Calories: 55 kcal
- Protein: 2g
- Carbohydrates: 12g
- Dietary Fiber: 2g
- Sugars: 0g
- Fat: 0.5g

EXERCISE FOR ENDOMORPHS

Endomorphs typically have a slower metabolism and may find it easier to gain weight, especially in the form of body fat. However, this doesn't mean they can't achieve their fitness goals. For endomorphs, it's essential to focus on exercises that promote fat loss while also building lean muscle mass.

1. **Cardiovascular Exercise**: Endomorphs benefit greatly from cardiovascular exercises that help burn calories and improve heart health. Activities like jogging, cycling, swimming, and HIIT (High-Intensity Interval Training) can be effective in burning excess calories and boosting metabolism.

2. **Strength Training**: Incorporating strength training into the workout routine is crucial for endomorphs. Lifting weights or doing bodyweight exercises helps build muscle mass, which in turn increases metabolic rate and aids in burning more calories even at rest.

3. **Compound Movements**: Exercises that target multiple muscle groups simultaneously are ideal for endomorphs. Compound movements like squats, deadlifts, lunges, and bench presses not only build strength but also help burn more calories compared to isolation exercises.

4. **Interval Training**: High-intensity interval training (HIIT) is particularly effective for endomorphs because it elevates the heart rate and burns a significant amount of calories in a shorter period. HIIT sessions can be customized to include both cardiovascular and strength-building exercises.

5. **Flexibility Training**: Endomorphs shouldn't overlook flexibility training. Incorporating activities like yoga or Pilates not only improves flexibility and mobility but also aids in stress reduction and overall well-being.

IMPORTANCE OF CONSISTENCY

Consistency is key for endomorphs (and for anyone pursuing fitness goals). Without consistency, it's challenging to see meaningful progress. Here's why consistency matters:

- **Progress Tracking:** Consistent exercise allows endomorphs to track their progress accurately. Whether it's weight loss, muscle gain, or improved endurance, consistency makes it easier to measure results over time.
- **Habit Formation:** Regular exercise helps establish a habit. Once exercise becomes a routine part of daily life, it's easier to stick to it long-term.
- **Metabolic Adaptation:** Consistent exercise helps the body adapt and become more efficient at burning calories and building muscle. Over time, this leads to better metabolic health and improved body composition.
- **Mental Benefits:** Exercise is not only beneficial for physical health but also for mental well-being. Consistent physical activity can reduce stress, anxiety, and depression, leading to a better overall quality of life.
- **Long-Term Sustainability:** Consistency fosters a sustainable approach to fitness. Rather than relying on short-term fixes or crash diets, consistent exercise promotes long-term health and fitness goals.

BALANCING CARDIO AND STRENGTH TRAINING

Balancing cardiovascular exercise with strength training is essential for endomorphs to achieve optimal results. Here's how to strike the right balance:

- **Prioritize Strength Training:** While cardiovascular exercise is important for calorie burning, endomorphs should prioritize strength training to build lean muscle mass. Muscle tissue burns more calories at rest than fat tissue, contributing to a higher metabolism.
- **Include Both in Your Routine:** Aim for a mix of cardiovascular exercise and strength training throughout the week. This could involve alternating days for each type of workout or incorporating both into a single session.
- **Customize Intensity:** The intensity of cardiovascular and strength workouts can be customized based on individual fitness levels and goals. High-intensity interval training (HIIT) can be particularly effective for combining cardio and strength benefits in one session.
- **Listen to Your Body:** Pay attention to how your body responds to different types of exercise. Some endomorphs may find they need more recovery time between intense cardio sessions, while others may thrive on a higher frequency of strength training.
- **Periodization:** Periodizing your training program by alternating between phases of higher cardio focus and higher strength focus can prevent plateaus and promote continuous progress.

REST AND RECOVERY

Rest and recovery are crucial components of any fitness program, especially for endomorphs who may be more prone to fatigue and muscle soreness. Here's why rest and recovery are important:

- **Muscle Repair and Growth:** Rest allows the body to repair and rebuild muscle tissue that's been broken down during exercise. This process is essential for muscle growth and strength development.
- **Prevention of Overtraining:** Overtraining can lead to decreased performance, increased risk of injury, and burnout. Rest days give the body time to recover and adapt to the stress of exercise.
- **Hormonal Balance:** Adequate rest helps maintain hormonal balance, which is essential for regulating metabolism, mood, and energy levels.
- **Injury Prevention:** Continuous exercise without sufficient rest increases the risk of overuse injuries. Taking regular rest days and incorporating active recovery activities like yoga or walking can reduce this risk.
- **Mental Well-being:** Rest is not just about physical recovery; it's also about mental rejuvenation. Taking breaks from intense workouts allows endomorphs to recharge mentally and stay motivated in the long run.

In summary, exercise for endomorphs should focus on a combination of cardiovascular exercise and strength training, with an emphasis on consistency, proper recovery, and individualized programming.

LIST OF EXERCISES

The key for endomorphs is a combination of cardiovascular exercise to burn fat and strength training to build and maintain muscle. Here is a list of exercises suitable for endomorphs along with instructions on how to perform them:

CARDIOVASCULAR EXERCISES

1. **Running or Jogging**
   - **How to perform:** Start with a warm-up of brisk walking or light jogging for 5-10 minutes. Then, increase your speed to a comfortable running pace. Maintain good posture, keeping your back straight and your shoulders relaxed. Aim to run for at least 20-30 minutes.
2. **Cycling**
   - **How to perform:** Use a stationary bike or a regular bicycle. Begin with a warm-up at a low resistance for 5-10 minutes. Increase the resistance or speed gradually. Maintain a steady pace for 30-45 minutes.
3. **Swimming**
   - **How to perform:** Start with a few minutes of easy swimming to warm up. Choose a stroke that you are comfortable with, such as freestyle or breaststroke. Swim continuously for 20-30 minutes, taking breaks if needed.
4. **High-Intensity Interval Training (HIIT)**
   - **How to perform:** Alternate between short bursts of intense activity (e.g., sprinting for 30 seconds) and periods of lower intensity (e.g., walking for 1 minute). Repeat for 20-30 minutes.

STRENGTH TRAINING EXERCISES

1. **Squats**
   - **How to perform:** Stand with your feet shoulder-width apart. Lower your body as if you are sitting in a chair, keeping your back straight and knees over your toes. Go as low as you can without losing form, then return to the starting position. Do 3 sets of 12-15 reps.

2. **Deadlifts**
   - **How to perform:** Stand with feet hip-width apart. Bend at your hips and knees to grab a barbell with an overhand grip. Keep your back straight and lift the barbell by straightening your hips and knees. Lower the bar back to the ground. Do 3 sets of 10-12 reps.

3. **Push-Ups**
   - **How to perform:** Start in a plank position with hands slightly wider than shoulder-width apart. Lower your body until your chest nearly touches the floor, keeping your elbows at a 45-degree angle. Push back up to the starting position. Do 3 sets of 10-15 reps.

4. **Pull-Ups**
   - **How to perform:** Grab a pull-up bar with an overhand grip, hands shoulder-width apart. Pull your body up until your chin is above the bar. Lower back down to the starting position. If you can't do a full pull-up, use an assisted pull-up machine or resistance bands. Do 3 sets of as many reps as possible.

5. **Plank**
   - **How to perform:** Lie face down on the floor. Lift your body up on your toes and forearms, keeping your body in a straight line from head to heels. Hold this position for as long as possible, aiming for at least 30 seconds. Do 3 sets.

FLEXIBILITY AND MOBILITY EXERCISES

1. **Yoga**
   - **How to perform:** Follow a yoga routine that includes poses like Downward Dog, Warrior Poses, and Child's Pose. Focus on breathing and holding each pose for several breaths. Aim for a 20-30 minute session.
2. **Dynamic Stretching**
   - **How to perform:** Perform movements that take your muscles through their full range of motion, such as leg swings, arm circles, and lunges with a twist. Do this as part of your warm-up for 5-10 minutes.

TIPS FOR SUCCESS

- **Consistency:** Regular exercise is key for endomorphs. Aim for at least 150 minutes of moderate-intensity or 75 minutes of high-intensity exercise each week.
- **Diet:** Complement your exercise routine with a balanced diet rich in whole foods, lean proteins, and plenty of vegetables. Control portion sizes to manage caloric intake.
- **Rest:** Ensure you get enough rest and recovery. Aim for 7-9 hours of sleep per night and include rest days in your exercise routine.

By combining these exercises with a healthy diet and adequate rest, endomorphs can effectively manage their weight and improve their overall fitness.

28-DAY EXERCISE PLAN

WEEK 1

Monday

- Warm-Up: Dynamic stretching (5 minutes)
- Cardio: Running or Jogging (20 minutes)
- Strength: Squats (3 sets of 12 reps)
- Cool Down: Static stretching (5 minutes)

Tuesday

Warm-Up: Dynamic stretching (5 minutes)

Strength: Push-Ups (3 sets of 10 reps)

Strength: Deadlifts (3 sets of 10 reps)

Cool Down: Static stretching (5 minutes)

Wednesday

- Rest Day or Light Activity: Yoga or a 30-minute walk

Thursday

Warm-Up: Dynamic stretching (5 minutes)

Cardio: Cycling (30 minutes)

Strength: Pull-Ups (3 sets of as many reps as possible)

Cool Down: Static stretching (5 minutes)

Friday

- Warm-Up: Dynamic stretching (5 minutes)
- Strength: Squats (3 sets of 12 reps)
- Strength: Plank (3 sets, hold for 30 seconds)
- Cool Down: Static stretching (5 minutes)

Saturday

Warm-Up: Dynamic stretching (5 minutes)

Cardio: Swimming (20 minutes)

Cool Down: Static stretching (5 minutes)

Sunday

- Rest Day or Light Activity: Yoga or a 30-minute walk

WEEK 2

Monday

- Warm-Up: Dynamic stretching (5 minutes)
- Cardio: Running or Jogging (25 minutes)
- Strength: Squats (3 sets of 15 reps)
- Cool Down: Static stretching (5 minutes)

Tuesday

Warm-Up: Dynamic stretching (5 minutes)

Strength: Push-Ups (3 sets of 12 reps)

Strength: Deadlifts (3 sets of 12 reps)

Cool Down: Static stretching (5 minutes)

Wednesday

- Rest Day or Light Activity: Yoga or a 30-minute walk

Thursday

Warm-Up: Dynamic stretching (5 minutes)

Cardio: Cycling (35 minutes)

Strength: Pull-Ups (3 sets of as many reps as possible)

Cool Down: Static stretching (5 minutes)

Friday

- Warm-Up: Dynamic stretching (5 minutes)
- Strength: Squats (3 sets of 15 reps)
- Strength: Plank (3 sets, hold for 35 seconds)
- Cool Down: Static stretching (5 minutes)

Saturday

Warm-Up: Dynamic stretching (5 minutes)

Cardio: Swimming (25 minutes)

Cool Down: Static stretching (5 minutes)

Sunday

- Rest Day or Light Activity: Yoga or a 30-minute walk

Monday

- Warm-Up: Dynamic stretching (5 minutes)
- Cardio: Running or Jogging (30 minutes)
- Strength: Squats (3 sets of 15 reps)
- Cool Down: Static stretching (5 minutes)

Tuesday

Warm-Up: Dynamic stretching (5 minutes)

Strength: Push-Ups (3 sets of 15 reps)

Strength: Deadlifts (3 sets of 12 reps)

Cool Down: Static stretching (5 minutes)

Wednesday

- Rest Day or Light Activity: Yoga or a 30-minute walk

Thursday

Warm-Up: Dynamic stretching (5 minutes)

Cardio: Cycling (40 minutes)

Strength: Pull-Ups (3 sets of as many reps as possible)

Cool Down: Static stretching (5 minutes)

Friday

- Warm-Up: Dynamic stretching (5 minutes)
- Strength: Squats (3 sets of 15 reps)
- Strength: Plank (3 sets, hold for 40 seconds)
- Cool Down: Static stretching (5 minutes)

Saturday

Warm-Up: Dynamic stretching (5 minutes)

Cardio: Swimming (30 minutes)

Cool Down: Static stretching (5 minutes)

Sunday

- Rest Day or Light Activity: Yoga or a 30-minute walk

WEEK 4

Monday

- Warm-Up: Dynamic stretching (5 minutes)
- Cardio: Running or Jogging (35 minutes)
- Strength: Squats (3 sets of 15 reps)
- Cool Down: Static stretching (5 minutes)

Tuesday

Warm-Up: Dynamic stretching (5 minutes)

Strength: Push-Ups (3 sets of 15 reps)

Strength: Deadlifts (3 sets of 12 reps)

Cool Down: Static stretching (5 minutes)

Wednesday

- Rest Day or Light Activity: Yoga or a 30-minute walk

Thursday

Warm-Up: Dynamic stretching (5 minutes)

Cardio: HIIT (20 minutes)

Strength: Pull-Ups (3 sets of as many reps as possible)

Cool Down: Static stretching (5 minutes)

Friday

- Warm-Up: Dynamic stretching (5 minutes)
- Strength: Squats (3 sets of 15 reps)
- Strength: Plank (3 sets, hold for 45 seconds)
- Cool Down: Static stretching (5 minutes)

Saturday

Warm-Up: Dynamic stretching (5 minutes)

Cardio: Swimming (35 minutes)

Cool Down: Static stretching (5 minutes)

Sunday

- Rest Day or Light Activity: Yoga or a 30-minute walk

NOTE:

NOTE:

NOTE:

NOTE: